Coping with Radiotherapy

TERRY PRIESTMAN is consultant clinical oncologist working at New Cross Hospital, Wolverhampton. He is also medical reviewer for the charity Cancerbackup (which provides information for cancer patients, their relatives and health professionals). He is a past Dean of the faculty of Clinical Oncology at the Royal College of Radiologists, and has written more than a hundred papers in the medical press. He is also the author of *Coping with Chemotherapy* (Sheldon Press, 2005) and *Coping with Breast Cancer* (Sheldon Press, 2006).

Overcoming Common Problems Series

Selected titles

A full list of titles is available from Sheldon Press,
36 Causton Street, London SW1P 4ST and on our website at
www.sheldonpress.co.uk

Assertiveness: Step by Step
Dr Windy Dryden and Daniel Constantinou

Breaking Free
Carolyn Ainscough and Kay Toon

Calm Down
Paul Hauck

Cataract: What You Need to Know
Mark Watts

Cider Vinegar
Margaret Hills

Comfort for Depression
Janet Horwood

Confidence Works
Gladeana McMahon

Coping Successfully with Pain
Neville Shone

Coping Successfully with Panic Attacks
Shirley Trickett

Coping Successfully with Period Problems
Mary-Claire Mason

Coping Successfully with Prostate Cancer
Dr Tom Smith

Coping Successfully with Ulcerative Colitis
Peter Cartwright

Coping Successfully with Your Hiatus Hernia
Dr Tom Smith

Coping Successfully with Your Irritable Bowel
Rosemary Nicol

Coping with Alopecia
Dr Nigel Hunt and Dr Sue McHale

Coping with Age-related Memory Loss
Dr Tom Smith

Coping with Blushing
Dr Robert Edelmann

Coping with Bowel Cancer
Dr Tom Smith

Coping with Brain Injury
Maggie Rich

Coping with Candida
Shirley Trickett

Coping with Chemotherapy
Dr Terry Priestman

Coping with Childhood Allergies
Jill Eckersley

Coping with Childhood Asthma
Jill Eckersley

Coping with Chronic Fatigue
Trudie Chalder

Coping with Coeliac Disease
Karen Brody

Coping with Cystitis
Caroline Clayton

Coping with Depression and Elation
Patrick McKeon

Coping with Down's Syndrome
Fiona Marshall

Coping with Dyspraxia
Jill Eckersley

Coping with Eating Disorders and Body Image
Christine Craggs-Hinton

Coping with Eczema
Dr Robert Youngson

Coping with Endometriosis
Jo Mears

Coping with Epilepsy
Fiona Marshall and Dr Pamela Crawford

Coping with Gout
Christine Craggs-Hinton

Coping with Hearing Loss
Christine Craggs-Hinton

Coping with Heartburn and Reflux
Dr Tom Smith

Coping with Incontinence
Dr Joan Gomez

Coping with Macular Degeneration
Dr Patricia Gilbert

Overcoming Common Problems Series

Coping with the Menopause
Janet Horwood

Coping with a Mid-life Crisis
Derek Milne

Coping with Polycystic Ovary Syndrome
Christine Craggs-Hinton

Coping with Postnatal Depression
Sandra L. Wheatley

Coping with SAD
Fiona Marshall and Peter Cheevers

Coping with Snoring and Sleep Apnoea
Jill Eckersley

Coping with a Stressed Nervous System
Dr Kenneth Hambly and Alice Muir

Coping with Strokes
Dr Tom Smith

Coping with Suicide
Maggie Helen

Coping with Thyroid Problems
Dr Joan Gomez

Depressive Illness
Dr Tim Cantopher

Eating for a Healthy Heart
Robert Povey, Jacqui Morrell and Rachel Povey

Effortless Exercise
Dr Caroline Shreeve

Fertility
Julie Reid

Free Your Life from Fear
Jenny Hare

Getting a Good Night's Sleep
Fiona Johnston

Heal the Hurt: How to Forgive and Move On
Dr Ann Macaskill

Help Your Child Get Fit Not Fat
Jan Hurst and Sue Hubberstey

Helping Children Cope with Anxiety
Jill Eckersley

Helping Children Cope with Change and Loss
Rosemary Wells

How to Approach Death
Julia Tugendhat

How to Be a Healthy Weight
Philippa Pigache

How to Be Your Own Best Friend
Dr Paul Hauck

How to Beat Pain
Christine Craggs-Hinton

How to Cope with Bulimia
Dr Joan Gomez

How to Cope with Difficult People
Alan Houel and Christian Godefroy

How to Improve Your Confidence
Dr Kenneth Hambly

How to Keep Your Cholesterol in Check
Dr Robert Povey

How to Make Life Happen
Gladeana McMahon

How to Stick to a Diet
Deborah Steinberg and Dr Windy Dryden

How to Stop Worrying
Dr Frank Tallis

How to Succeed in Psychometric Tests
David Cohen

How to Talk to Your Child
Penny Oates

Hysterectomy
Suzie Hayman

Is HRT Right for You?
Dr Anne MacGregor

Letting Go of Anxiety and Depression
Dr Windy Dryden

Living with Alzheimer's Disease
Dr Tom Smith

Living with Asperger Syndrome
Dr Joan Gomez

Living with Asthma
Dr Robert Youngson

Living with Autism
Fiona Marshall

Living with Crohn's Disease
Dr Joan Gomez

Living with Fibromyalgia
Christine Craggs-Hinton

Living with Food Intolerance
Alex Gazzola

Living with Grief
Dr Tony Lake

Living with Heart Failure
Susan Elliot-Wright

Living with Hughes Syndrome
Triona Holden

Overcoming Common Problems Series

Overcoming Common Problems

Coping with Radiotherapy

DR TERRY PRIESTMAN

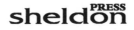

First published in Great Britain in 2007

Sheldon Press
36 Causton Street
London SW1P 4ST

British Library Cataloguing-in-Publication Data
A catalogue record for this book is available from the British Library

ISBN 978-0-85969-999-0

1 3 5 7 9 10 8 6 4 2

Typeset by Fakenham Photosetting Ltd, Fakenham, Norfolk
Printed in Great Britain by Ashford Colour Press

Contents

Introduction

Understanding radiotherapy

Radiotherapy is one of the most high-tech areas of modern-day medicine, with amazingly complicated treatment machines, and the most sophisticated of computers, being used in the delivery of the radiation. People sometimes worry that all this technology might mean that their treatment will be cold and impersonal, supervised and carried out by staff who are more interested in their machines than their patients. Nothing could be further from the truth. Radiotherapy is one of the most human areas of medicine, as people with cancer are among the most frightened and vulnerable of all patients, and helping them cope with their illness, and very often being able to cure them completely, is the real reason that your treatment team has chosen to work in this branch of medicine.

Becoming a specialist doctor in giving radiotherapy takes years of training. In England and Wales at the moment there are about 125,000 doctors, of whom less than 500 are qualified to give radiotherapy. Because it has been considered such a specialized field, most doctors, including general practitioners and other hospital consultants, will have little or no training in, or experience of, radiotherapy. This is despite the fact that about one in eight of us will have treatment with radiotherapy at some time during our lives.

This relative lack of knowledge of many clinicians, combined with a widespread public suspicion of anything to do with radiation and radioactivity, added to some people's family memories of relatives who suffered side effects from the relatively crude types of radiotherapy treatment that was all that was available some forty or so years ago, mean that myths and misunderstandings about this potentially life-saving treatment abound. So very often, when someone is told they will need radiotherapy, the news stirs up all kinds of fears and uncertainties, which are often compounded by well-meant misinformation from family, friends and even health professionals. In the coming chapters I hope we will be able to demystify this vital form of treatment, which improves the outcome for so many people who have cancer.

So what is radiotherapy? Radiotherapy is the use of ionizing radiation to treat disease.

This sentence needs a bit of explaining. Radiation is a way of carrying energy in the form of either electromagnetic waves or invisible particles. Radio waves, microwaves, light waves, ultraviolet rays and X-rays are some of the different types of radiation energy. These various types of radiation are divided into two groups, ionizing and non-ionizing. Ionizing radiations carry more energy than non-ionizing radiations. In fact they carry so much energy that they cause changes in the atoms of anything they meet. These changes are called ionization and are explained a bit more in Chapter 5. Non-ionizing radiations are weaker rays that don't cause ionization.

Radio waves, microwaves, light waves and infrared rays are all non-ionizing types of radiation. Ionizing radiations may be either electromagnetic waves, like X-rays or gamma rays, or may take the form of particles, like electrons, neutrons and protons. Ionizing radiation can occur naturally or be man-made. Natural ionizing radiation comes from four main sources:

- *cosmic radiation*, coming from deep space, beyond our solar system;
- *solar radiation*, coming from the sun;
- *geological radiation*, coming from traces of radioactive chemicals in the rocks that make up the earth's surface;
- *radon gas*, which is radioactive and is present in small traces in the air around us.

All of us are constantly exposed to minute amounts of ionizing radiation from these natural sources. In fact in the UK the dose of ionizing radiation we get from nature is about 55,000 times more than the dose we get from pollution due to the nuclear fuel industry. Even so, these doses of natural radiation are far too small to cause us any harm. The nuclear fuel industry is one example of man-made ionizing radiation, and nuclear weapons are another.

The different types of rays and particles used in radiotherapy are also man-made ionizing radiations.

When someone is exposed to ionizing radiation there will be ionization changes in the cells of whichever part of their body has been irradiated. If the radiation is given at too high a dose then these changes can be very damaging, but if it is given in a carefully controlled way then it can actually help in the treatment of a number of diseases.

These days, radiotherapy is usually only used to treat cancer. But in the past it has also been given as part of the treatment of some benign (non-cancerous) illnesses, and is still occasionally used in this way.

Radiotherapy and chemotherapy

When they are going to have treatment for a cancer some people do get confused between radiotherapy and chemotherapy.

Chemotherapy means the use of drugs to treat an illness. So when we talk about cancer chemotherapy we simply mean using drugs to treat the cancer. These days a wide variety of anti-cancer drugs is available, and the number is increasing all the time. Until very recently the two main groups of anti-cancer drugs have been the cytotoxics and hormones. Cytotoxics are cell poisons; they cause damage, and death, to cancer cells (they can also damage normal cells, which is why they may cause troublesome side effects like sickness and hair loss). Cytotoxics are used as part of the treatment of a wide range of different types of cancer. Hormone drugs are used mainly as part of the treatment of either breast or prostate cancer, where the tumours often need certain hormones to drive their growth, and giving drugs that change the balance of hormones in the body can slow them down, so that they shrink or even disappear. More recently other types of drugs have been developed that can attack cancers in different ways. These include the monoclonal antibodies (like Herceptin, which may help some women with breast cancer, and Avastin that may help some people with bowel cancer) and drugs that attack the chemical messengers that cause a cancer cell to multiply (like Glivec, which is useful for some people with chronic leukaemia).

So the range of drugs that can be used in cancer chemotherapy is increasing all the time. (For more information, see Dr Terry Priestman, *Coping with Chemotherapy*, Sheldon Press, 2005.)

These chemotherapy drugs may be given as tablets or injections or infusions (drips) into a vein. Radiotherapy is most often given by using machines that produce a beam of radiation that is focused on the cancer.

So radiotherapy and chemotherapy are completely different types of treatment. The other main type of treatment used against cancer is surgery. Different cancers are treated in different ways. Sometimes surgery, using an operation to take the cancer away, is all that is needed, less commonly radiotherapy or chemotherapy may be the only treatments necessary. But these days treatment for a cancer usually involves a combination of two or more different approaches, often combining surgery, radiotherapy and chemotherapy to give the best chance of a cure.

Local and general treatment

An important difference between radiotherapy and chemotherapy is that one is a local treatment and the other is a general treatment.

If you have a dose of chemotherapy, whether as a tablet, an injection or an infusion, the drug that is given will find its way into your bloodstream and will be carried throughout your body. A treatment that affects most parts of the body in this way is sometimes called a systemic treatment. So cancer chemotherapy is a systemic therapy.

By contrast, radiotherapy is almost always targeted to a particular part of the body where the cancer is present. It acts just on that one area, and so is a local treatment (like surgery, which is also a local treatment, simply removing a block of tissue or a particular organ).

As we will see in more detail later, this difference between local and general, or systemic, effects of the different treatments is important in understanding both the reasons why they are given and the side effects they may cause.

1

A bit of history

On the evening of 8 November 1895, Conrad Röntgen discovered X-rays. Like so many scientific and medical discoveries it was something of an accident, which came about while he was researching cathode rays (which years later were to be crucial in the development of television). Röntgen noticed that rays from one of his cathode tubes illuminated a paper plate covered with barium salts, and that when his wife put her hand in the beam of those rays it produced a picture of the bones of her fingers on the plate – the first X-ray.

Within days of reporting his discovery, on 1 January 1896, other people were busy taking X-ray pictures of everything they could lay there hands on, and beginning to realize that they might help to identify and diagnose disease. The speed with which these same rays were considered as a possibility for treating illnesses was in part due to the fact that what seemed to be a similar approach to treatment was already in widespread use. Since the discovery of electricity, electrotherapy had flourished during the Victorian era. All manner of weird and wonderful machines were invented to deliver small, or sometimes quite large, doses of electricity to willing patients who were encouraged to believe that the tingles and shocks they experienced as a result would help cure their ailments. Of the countless devices used, one North American machine claimed to cure everything from arthritis to insomnia, constipation, obesity and, of course, cancer.

Adapting this existing technology to make the first crude X-ray machines was relatively easy, and a public widely familiar with the supposed benefits of electrotherapy was happy to embrace the novelty of what seemed to be simply a new version of that treatment. The credit for who actually gave the first radiotherapy treatment, with X-rays, is still hotly disputed. Many Americans favour Emil Grubbé, an electrotherapist in Chicago, who claimed that within a month of Röntgen's initial announcement of his discovery he began treating a woman called Rose Lee for advanced breast cancer with X-rays. However, as no record of that treatment, which supposedly began on 29 January 1896, exists, and as it was not until more than thirty-five years later that Grubbé made his claim, many people doubt his assertion – a doubt reinforced by his biographer's description of him as 'vain, boastful and incompletely truthful'.

On the other side of the Atlantic the honour of being the founding father of radiotherapy is claimed for at least two individuals: Victor Despeignes in France and Leopold Freund in Austria. Despeignes' treatment of a man with stomach cancer, in July 1896, is well documented. But the equipment he used would have produced such weak X-rays that they really could have had no effect, and although a brief benefit was claimed, the patient died within ten days of treatment. Freund's patient was a 5-year-old girl with a benign (non-cancerous) skin condition. Photographs show her improvement, although with a lot of skin damage from the radiation at the time, and she was alive 80 years later when further photographs showed her condition had been cured, although she had quite severe scarring of her skin from the original treatment.

Whoever one credits with their introduction as a new form of therapy the use of X-ray beams to treat illness rapidly became accepted by the medical profession. Reports of the first definite cures of cancer were published in 1900 (two people with skin cancer, treated in Sweden), and the first textbook on the subject came out a year later.

A year after Röntgen made his discovery of X-rays, the Frenchman Henri Becquerel discovered natural ionizing radiation, when he found that uranium salts affected photographic plates in a similar way to X-rays. Two years later, in 1898, Marie and Pierre Curie discovered the radioactive element radium. Like the uranium salts this produced beams of ionizing radiation, although these were beams of γ (gamma) rays, rather than X-rays.

Over the following decades radiotherapy developed in several directions. The original primitive electrotherapy-based equipment for producing X-rays became increasingly sophisticated, evolving through a series of machines with names straight out of science fiction, like orthovoltage units, van der Graaf generators and betatrons. The breakthrough came in the early 1950s with the virtually simultaneous introduction in California and London, in 1952 and 1953 respectively, of the first linear accelerators. These high-energy machines were able to produce beams of radiation that could penetrate deep into the tissues of the body with great accuracy, and with little or no damage to the skin. Over the last fifty years linear accelerators have become increasingly complex and versatile but they are the still the machines that underpin more than nine out of ten of today's radiotherapy treatments.

The use of radioactive elements like radium, and later cobalt, to produce γ ray beams allowed a different type of radiotherapy machine to be produced, culminating in the early 1950s in the first cobalt treatment unit in London, Ontario, in 1951, and rather dramatically named the cobalt bomb. These radioactive elements could also be used in another way. They were made into needles, wires or other shapes that could be inserted directly into cancers, or placed up against them, giving intense doses of local, short-distance radiation rather than producing a beam from a machine.

Although the possible benefits of radiotherapy in treating cancer were rapidly recognized, the potential dangers also became apparent quite quickly. In Hamburg in 1902 the first case of skin cancer caused by X-rays was diagnosed in a man who worked with X-ray tubes. Despite this, the real hazards of the new X and γ radiations were not fully appreciated for some years. As a result, many pioneers in the field, both those working with the radiation and those treated by it, went on to develop skin cancers or leukaemia some years later because of the uncontrolled doses that were given. In fact, in Hamburg a monument was erected in 1936, commemorating 170 people who had died from these radiation-related injuries.

As a result of these early disasters enormous progress was made in radiation protection and the safe delivery of radiotherapy, so that nowadays the benefits vastly outweigh any risks associated with the treatment. One hundred years on, radiotherapy is as safe, or safer, than most other forms of treatment.

At first, radiotherapy services in the UK developed in a rather haphazard way, but in 1929 the National Radium Trust and Radium Commission was established to oversee the purchase of radium and its use in cancer treatment. The Commission decided on a number of hospitals to develop local radiotherapy services. There were eight of these in England (London, Birmingham, Bristol, Leeds, Liverpool, Manchester, Newcastle and Sheffield), four in Scotland (Aberdeen, Dundee, Edinburgh and Glasgow) and one each in Wales and Northern Ireland (Cardiff and Belfast). The Cancer Act of 1938 told local authorities to develop cancer services, but this work was largely interrupted by the war and was then taken over by the newly formed NHS in 1948. Radiotherapy services have steadily expanded and there are now 57 hospitals throughout the UK where radiotherapy is given. This still means that many people will not have a radiotherapy department in their local hospital, and will have to travel some distance for treatment. Unfortunately, because the equipment needed to deliver radiotherapy is so expensive, and because it requires specially trained teams of staff, it is only possible to have the service at a limited number of hospitals across the UK.

2

How is radiotherapy given?

Radiotherapy can be given in a number of different ways. These can be grouped into three types of treatment called teletherapy, brachytherapy and radio-isotope therapy.

Teletherapy

Teletherapy is also known as external beam therapy, and this gives a better idea of what is actually involved. In this type of treatment the patient lies on a couch under a machine that produces a beam of ionizing radiation. That beam of radiation is directed at the part of the body where the treatment needs to be given. The radiation beam is invisible, and doesn't cause any feeling or sensation (just like an ordinary chest X-ray, where you don't see or feel anything when the X-ray picture is taken).

Although the machines that deliver the treatment are often very complex, and the planning that goes on before the treatment starts is frequently very sophisticated, the actual treatment itself, from the patient's point of view, is incredibly simple – just a matter of lying still for a few moments at a time. No pain, no tingling or burning, no injections or tablets, and no immediate side effects (and often no side effects at all). You feel no different when you walk out of the room after your treatment session from how you did when you walked in.

As the treatment beam is made up of ionizing radiation, it is 'radioactive'. But once the treatment machine is switched off, at the end of your session, the beam disappears, and so does the radioactivity. So you are not radioactive after your treatment – you don't store up any radiation inside you – it is perfectly safe to mix with family and friends after your treatment visit, and you certainly won't glow in the dark!

Although you are not radioactive before or after your treatment, while you are lying on the couch and the machine is switched on it is giving out a beam of ionizing radiation. Although this beam is focused on the part of you that has to be treated, tiny amounts of that radiation will be scattered throughout the room. The scattered radiation is of such low intensity that it will do you no harm for the few minutes you are having your treatment. But if the staff who are giving you your treatment (the therapy radiographers) stayed in the room with you then, with up to 50 people being treated each day, over time they would build up a dangerous level of exposure from the scattered radiation. This is why you have to be in the treatment room on your own when the radiotherapy machine is switched on. Your radiographers will be with you before and after your treatment, but while you are actually having your radiotherapy they will be at their control desk, immediately outside the room, watching you on CCTV. They will be able to see and hear you, so if you are worried at any time during your treatment you can wave or call and they will stop the machine and come in to help you.

External beam therapy is used for the great majority of radiation treatments. About 95 out of every 100 people who have radiotherapy will have this type of treatment.

Brachytherapy

In this approach to treatment a source of ionizing radiation is placed close to, or actually inside, a cancer. The two conditions where brachytherapy is most often used nowadays are cancer of the cervix (the neck of the womb) and prostate cancer.

When brachytherapy is used as part of the treatment of a cervical cancer it involves a short stay in hospital. The treatment pathway begins by going to an operating theatre and having a general anaesthetic. But there is no operation. What happens is that after a thorough pelvic examination, to check the size and position of the cancer, three hollow metal tubes are carefully slipped into the vagina, rather like putting in a tampon (see Figures 1a and 1b). The tubes are placed around the cancer and, once the specialist thinks they are in the right position, gauze bandages are packed around them, in the vagina, so that they stay in place. The ends of the tube, which stick out from the vagina, are fixed by a special

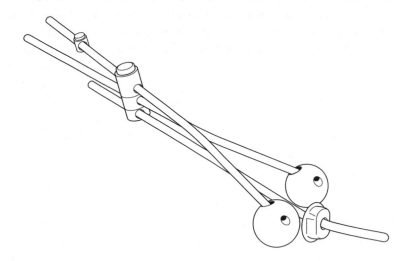

Figure 1a The hollow tubes (applicators) used to place radioactive sources for treatment of gynaecological cancers

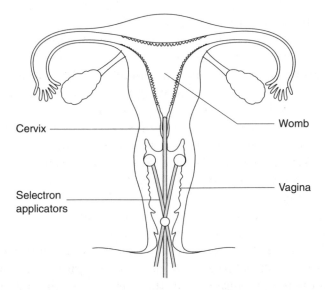

Figure 1b Applicators in place for treatment of a cancer of the cervix

clamp, which also helps make sure they don't move. The patient is then taken back to a special room on the ward. The ends of the hollow tubes are then connected to a machine called a Selectron. The Selectron is specially programmed, and when it is switched on it sends a number of small pellets of radioactive material down the tubes, so that these come to lie in the end of the tubes, around the cancer. These pellets give off very intense ionizing radiation around the cancer and the cervix, but the radiation only penetrates a very short distance, so nearby normal tissues are relatively unaffected, keeping side effects down.

The caesium pellets are radioactive, and this means that while they are in place around the cancer, the patient is radioactive as well. If a nurse or a visitor needs to spend some time with them, then the Selectron can be switched off and the pellets will go back into the machine, leaving everything perfectly safe. Once the visit is over the machine is switched back on, the pellets go back down the tubes and the treatment continues. Depending on the precise dose needed, the tubes may stay in place for anything from a matter of minutes up to a few days. Once the treatment is complete the Selectron is switched off for a final time and the metal tubes, and surrounding gauze packing, can easily be removed on the ward without the need for another anaesthetic.

In some centres higher intensity radioactive sources are used with a machine called a Microselectron. With this approach treatment times can be reduced to a matter of minutes, with several sessions being given over a few days. Although this means that the actual length of time when the radioactive sources are inside you is shorter, it can be more uncomfortable and may carry a slightly greater risk of complications. Because this treatment uses radioactive sources that are put into devices which have been placed in position by the cancer beforehand, this type of brachytherapy is sometimes called after-loading.

When brachytherapy is used to treat prostate cancer, the approach is rather different. Once again an anaesthetic is involved but this time a special instrument is used to put a number of metal seeds containing radioactive iodine into the prostate gland. The instrument may be pushed into the gland either through a small cut in the skin of the pelvis, or by slipping it into the back passage and through the wall of the bowel, which lies next to the prostate. These seeds then stay in the prostate permanently. Over the following weeks the radioactive iodine gives off intense irradiation to the tissue in the prostate gland, killing the cancer cells. Over time the radio-iodine decays and it loses its radioactive power. While the iodine is active it does mean that the patient will be radioactive but the radiation from the iodine only penetrates a tiny distance, and so will not affect other people; it is quite safe for the patient to mix with family and friends in a normal way.

There are other types of brachytherapy that may occasionally be used but these are the two commonest approaches, and they give an idea of the general principles of this type of radiotherapy. Overall brachytherapy probably makes up fewer than 5 out of every 100 radiation treatments in the UK, although it is more widely used in some other countries.

Systemic radio-isotope therapy

In this type of treatment a radioactive substance is introduced into the body, either as a capsule to be swallowed or as a fluid to be injected into a vein. In both cases the isotope then enters the bloodstream and circulates around the body. It is then concentrated in certain tissues or organs, which it irradiates. Once swallowed or injected the isotope cannot be removed, but it gradually decays and the level of radiation falls with time and eventually disappears.

Three types of radio-isotope are used: radioactive iodine, radioactive phosphorus, and radioactive strontium. Radio-iodine is used as part of the treatment of some types of thyroid cancer, and to treat the non-cancerous condition of an overactive thyroid gland (hyperthyroidism). This is because the body concentrates iodine in thyroid tissue, so after a capsule of radio-iodine is swallowed, the isotope will build up in the thyroid gland, with very little in other tissues. In a similar way, both radio-phosphorus, and radio-strontium are concentrated in the bones. Radio-phosphorus is used as one approach to treatment for a fairly uncommon condition called primary polycythaemia (polycythaemia rubra vera), where the bone marrow makes too many red blood cells. Radioactive strontium is sometimes used to treat cancer that has spread to the bones from a primary cancer somewhere else in the body (secondaries in the bone, sometimes called bone metastases).

The use of radio-isotopes in this way is a fairly uncommon type of treatment and fewer than 1 person in every 100 who has radiotherapy will have systemic radio-isotope therapy.

How is teletherapy given?

A number of different machines are used to deliver external beam radiotherapy. The main difference between these machines is the energy of the beam of radiation that they produce. The importance of beam energy is that the greater the energy, the deeper the beam will penetrate into the tissues; a higher-energy beam will go further into the body than a lower-energy beam. The main types of external beam radiotherapy machine in use today are superficial units, orthovoltage machines, cobalt units and linear accelerators (LinAcs).

Superficial units

These are very simple radiotherapy machines (see Figure 2). The heart of the machine is an X-ray tube, about 30–50 cm (12–18 inches) in length. All X-ray tubes work on the same principle of producing a beam made up of electrons which then hit a metal target; the interaction of the electrons and the target then produces the beam of X-rays.

The superficial unit comes with a range of applicators. One end of these is fitted to the X-ray tube, and the other rests against the patient's skin during treatment. The size of the applicator determines the size of the patch of skin which is irradiated. The beam produced by these units is of very low energy, and only penetrates a few millimetres into the skin. The deeper tissues are completely unaffected. This means that they are only suitable for treating certain types of skin cancer.

When it comes to skin cancers, most people have heard of malignant melanomas, but these only make up a minority of these tumours. The commonest type of skin cancer is called a basal cell carcinoma (these are also known as rodent ulcers); another quite common skin cancer is a squamous carcinoma. Basal cell

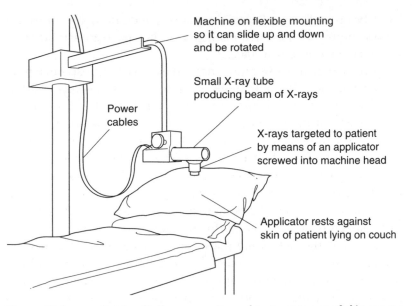

Machine on flexible mounting so it can slide up and down and be rotated

Small X-ray tube producing beam of X-rays

Power cables

X-rays targeted to patient by means of an applicator screwed into machine head

Applicator rests against skin of patient lying on couch

Figure 2 A superficial radiotherapy unit used to treat types of skin cancer

carcinomas and squamous skin carcinomas are often grouped together as non-melanomatous skin cancers. Each year in Britain about 8,000 new cases of malignant melanoma are diagnosed, but there are more than 100,000 new cases of the non-melanomatous skin cancers. So, basal and squamous cell cancers of the skin are a common problem.

The cornerstone of treatment for malignant melanoma is surgery, and radiotherapy plays little or no part. But basal and squamous cell skin cancers both respond very well to radiotherapy, and the great majority of them can be cured with a single treatment, given as an outpatient, and lasting about five minutes.

So although superficial units only produce a weak beam of radiation, and are restricted to treating non-melanomatous skin cancers, they are responsible for curing countless thousands of cancers every year in the UK.

Orthovoltage machines

Orthovoltage machines work on the same principle as superficial units but have a bigger, fatter X-ray tube, which produces a bigger, fatter beam of X-rays. These X-rays can penetrate deeper into the tissues but lose a lot of their energy once they have gone more than 10 cm below the skin surface.

Orthovoltage units were the major type of radiotherapy machine in the UK up until the mid-1960s. Because of the limited penetration of their beam it meant that if a cancer was being treated that lay quite deep within the body then a very high dose of radiation would have to be given to the skin in order to give anything like an effective dose to the cancer. As a result, patients being treated by these machines often developed severe skin damage: the skin would become red and sore, often blistering and peeling, and sometimes there would be permanent skin damage after treatment, with darkening of the skin, the formation of prominent blood vessels – making spidery red marks on the skin (which doctors call telangiectasia) – and sometimes quite severe scarring. As we will see, with modern day radiotherapy machines skin damage is seldom a problem, but many people have memories of parents or grand-parents who were treated 50 or 60 years ago and had terrible skin reactions after their radiotherapy. It is important to be reassured that the chances of bad skin damage from treatment nowadays are very small indeed.

Orthovoltage units are disappearing from radiotherapy centres in the UK but they may still be used occasionally, particularly in the treatment of some advanced cancers, where, among other things, they can help ease symptoms like bone pain, or ease the discomfort from enlarged lymph nodes that have become swollen by the presence of cancer cells.

Cobalt units

These first appeared in the early 1950s, with the first machine being installed in the Victoria Hospital in London, Ontario. They work on a completely different principle to other radiotherapy machines. Rather than using an X-ray tube, to produce X-rays, they rely on a pellet of radioactive cobalt, which is continually decaying to produce high-energy gamma rays. Gamma rays are another type of ionizing radiation.

Cobalt units are very simple. They consist of a thick protective metal shell that contains the pellet of radioactive cobalt (which is about the size of a thumbnail). In the side of this shell are a set of shutters; when these are opened then the beam of radiation from the cobalt escapes and irradiates the patient lying under the machine. The size of the beam is controlled by adjusting the width to which the shutters are opened.

In the UK and a large number of other countries cobalt units have all but disappeared, but in many parts of the world they are the mainstay of radiotherapy treatment. Although they are less versatile and do not produce such a high-energy beam as linear accelerators, they are adequate for treating many types of cancer, and have the advantages of being relatively cheap, technically simple, requiring little maintenance, and very reliable.

Linear accelerators

Linear accelerators (LinAcs) first appeared at about the same time as cobalt units, with the first machine coming into operation in Stanford, California, in 1952. Like superficial and orthovoltage units, LinAcs use a beam of electrons striking a metal target to produce their X-ray beam. But they are capable of generating beams with a far greater energy than those other machines. To put this in perspective, the energy of a radiation beam is measured in electron volts; superficial units produce beams with an energy of about 80,000–100,000 electron volts, orthovoltage units work in the range 180,000–350,000 electron volts, but LinAcs produce beams with energies between 4 and 20 million electron volts. (For completeness: the gamma ray beam produced by cobalt units has an energy of 1.3 million electron volts, and because both cobalt units and LinAcs generate beams with energies in excess of 1 million electron volts, they are sometimes called megavoltage machines.)

The very high-energy beam produced by modern-day LinAcs has at least three advantages:

1 the beam can penetrate very deeply into the tissues of the body without losing much of its energy;
2 even deep inside the body the beam remains sharp and precise, so it can be very accurately targeted to cancerous tissue;
3 radiation beams with energies greater than 1 million electron

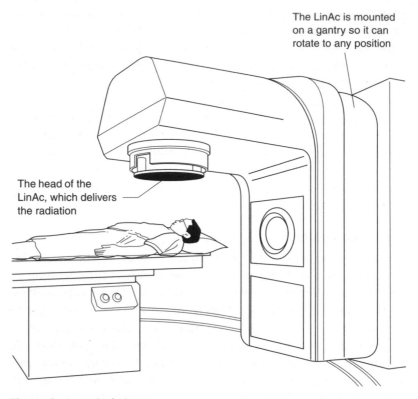

The LinAc is mounted on a gantry so it can rotate to any position

The head of the LinAc, which delivers the radiation

Figure 3   A typical LinAc

volts actually shoot through the first centimetre or two of tissue that they meet before they begin to irradiate. This means that they only begin to release their radiation energy below skin level. So they have a skin-sparing effect, and do not produce the same sort of skin damage that was seen with the orthovoltage machines.

LinAcs are mounted on a gantry which means they can rotate through a complete circle, so you can be treated from any position (see Figure 3). The head of the treatment machine has jaws, or shutters, which can open to different widths, and this controls the size of the beam reaching the patient. This can vary from as little as 1cm across to up to 40 cm or more. Some LinAcs have a special device which allows the metal target in the head of the machine to be slipped to one side, so that you can be treated by a beam of electrons, rather than X-rays. As we will see later, electron beams have a different pattern of absorption in the tissue to X-rays, which makes them particularly useful for some types of cancer.

The fact that LinAcs can rotate to different positions is very important because the best coverage of the cancer by the radiation is usually achieved by treating it with several beams from different directions. The beams intersect at the point where the cancer is, maximizing the dose to the growth and keeping the dose to normal tissue to a minimum (see Figure 4, page 47). From the patient's point of view, this means that when they have their treatment they lie on the couch to have their first dose of radiation. The LinAc rotates to a different angle and delivers a further dose from the new position. Depending on the site and size of the cancer being treated, anything from two to six different radiation beams might be used, but the patient lies still all the time while the LinAc moves to each of the new treatment positions.

In the UK, and most developed countries, LinAcs are now the principal way in which radiotherapy is delivered, and more than 90 out of every 100 people who have radiotherapy in Britain today will have their treatment on a LinAc.

3

Why do I need radiotherapy?

Radiotherapy can be used for a number of different reasons in cancer treatment. A few words about the way cancers grow and develop will help in understanding the different roles radiotherapy can play.

Most cancers begin as a few abnormal cells in one part of the body. Over a period of time, usually a number of years, these will gradually multiply to form a lump or swelling. This is called the primary cancer. If it is not treated this primary will carry on growing, and in time cells will break off from it and travel through either the lymph vessels or the bloodstream, and go to other parts of the body. These cancer seedlings will then grow to form secondary cancers, or metastases. To begin with, these secondaries will be made up of relatively few cancer cells and will be too small to see, or to show up on any scans or X-rays, but over time, which again may be a period of many months or even years, they will grow to form cancerous lumps that will cause symptoms and problems.

Just to give an example, if we think of a bowel cancer, this will start as a cancerous change in some cells in the lining of part of the large bowel (either the colon or rectum) and slowly grow to form a swelling or an ulcer in the wall of the bowel. This is the primary cancer. If this isn't removed by an operation, then with time the cancer will grow through the wall of the bowel into the surrounding tissues and send off seedlings of tumour into the nearby lymph nodes. Cells are also likely to go into the blood vessels and be carried to other organs, most often to the liver, but sometimes to the lungs and other places as well. These cells will grow to form secondary cancers in the lymph nodes, the liver and wherever else they lodge. These are secondary bowel cancers, made up of bowel cancer cells. So a secondary cancer in the liver from a primary cancer in the colon or rectum behaves like a bowel cancer, and will respond to the same treatment as the primary tumour. It is completely different from a primary cancer of the liver, which is a cancer that has started in the liver and not one that has spread from somewhere else in the body.

Cancer treatment

There are three main ways of treating cancer: surgery, radiotherapy and chemotherapy. (Some people use the word chemotherapy to describe just one type of treatment, known as cytotoxic therapy, but we will use it to cover all types of drug treatment for cancer.)

Surgery remains the cornerstone of treatment for primary cancers. Wherever possible an operation will be done to take away a primary cancer. But if that cancer is too big, or if it is in a part of the body where surgery might be dangerous, or if it has already spread to other places, then surgery may not be possible. Surgery, like most radiotherapy, is a local treatment, only affecting one part of the body. By contrast chemotherapy goes into the bloodstream and affects nearly all parts of the body. So it is a general or, to use the medical word, a systemic, treatment.

Each type of treatment has its strengths and weaknesses. Surgery is very good if a primary cancer is still quite small and hasn't spread. But it can't be used for big cancers, or when there are multiple secondary cancers in different parts of the body. Radiotherapy is good at treating some primary cancers, and can often cover a wider area of tissue than it would be safe to remove in an operation, and it can help ease symptoms from some secondary cancers. Chemotherapy is fairly ineffective against most primary cancers (although the haematological cancers, the leukaemias, lymphomas and myeloma are an exception to this rule), but has a valuable role in preventing or treating the secondary spread of a cancer.

One of the things that led to great improvements in cancer treatment during the latter part of the twentieth century was the realization that these different approaches to treatment (different treatment modalities) could be combined rather than used separately. So today someone might have an operation to remove their primary cancer, followed by radiotherapy and then chemotherapy in order to give them the best chance of a cure, rather than just having one type of treatment.

Given this background we can look at the different ways that radiotherapy might be used as part of a programme of cancer treatment.

Pre-operative therapy

If a surgeon feels that a primary cancer is just a bit too big to be successfully taken away by an operation, radiotherapy can sometimes be given to shrink the tumour and make an operation possible. The radiotherapy may be given on its own, or combined with chemotherapy.

Primary therapy

This is where radiotherapy is used as the first line of treatment to deal with a primary cancer. In some cancers radiotherapy is just as effective as surgery and it is a matter of patient choice as to which type of treatment is used. Both approaches will cause varying amounts of inconvenience and disruption, and will almost always have the risk of some side effects. The pros and cons of the different treatments should be clearly explained and then it is up to the individual to choose which option they would prefer as their therapy.

Sometimes an operation might normally be the best approach but the patient may not be fit enough to undergo major surgery. So for some older people, or people who have a lot of other medical problems apart from their cancer, radiotherapy might be a safer alternative.

Post-operative adjuvant therapy

Even when a surgeon feels that he or she has completely removed a primary cancer there is still sometimes the risk that invisible microscopic traces of the tumour might have been left behind. In time these could grow and form a local recurrence of the cancer. In this situation, giving a course of radiotherapy after surgery, covering the area where the tumour was and a generous margin of normal tissue roundabout, can greatly reduce the risk of a local recurrence developing.

Giving treatment to prevent the risk of secondary cancers growing from microscopic seedlings of cancer cells is called adjuvant therapy, and so this type of radiotherapy, given following an operation, is often called post-operative adjuvant therapy.

Preventive radiotherapy, prophylactic therapy

This is a relatively uncommon use of radiotherapy. It involves giving a course of treatment to a part of the body where doctors feel seedlings from a primary cancer might have spread, and it is intended to kill off those microscopic secondary cancers before they can grow to cause symptoms and problems.

Palliative therapy

This is treatment given when a cancer has reached a more advanced stage, and is no longer curable. However, either radiotherapy or chemotherapy can often do a great deal to ease unpleasant symptoms, and may also help people to live longer. This type of treatment, directed mainly at helping relieve things like pain, breathlessness, headache, bleeding or a cough, is known as palliative therapy.

Radiotherapy in the treatment of common cancers

The four commonest types of cancer in the UK are breast cancer, lung cancer, prostate cancer and bowel cancer. Radiotherapy can play a part in the treatment of all these tumours and we can use them as examples to show how and why radiation is used.

Breast cancer

In primary breast cancer the first line of treatment is almost always surgery, with removal of the lump from the breast, either by an operation to take away the cancer and a small margin of normal breast tissue, a lumpectomy, or by a bigger operation taking away the whole of the breast, a mastectomy. Radiotherapy is almost always given after a lumpectomy, and quite often after a mastectomy, in order to reduce the risk of the cancer coming back. Even if the breast cancer was small, and the surgeon was confident it had been completely removed, there is still about a one in three chance of a local recurrence; giving post-operative adjuvant radiotherapy greatly reduces this risk. This is the commonest use of radiotherapy in the UK, and the post-operative radiation of people who have had a breast cancer removed makes up a major part of the workload of all radiotherapy departments. Radiotherapy is not often given as a pre-operative, neoadjuvant treatment to shrink breast cancers; on the few occasions when neoadjuvant treatment is used it usually involves chemotherapy or hormone therapy.

Radiotherapy plays an important part in symptom control for people with advanced breast cancer and short courses of treatment, or even single doses of radiation, can do a lot to ease bone pain and other problems. (For more information, see Dr Terry Priestman, *Coping with Breast Cancer*, Sheldon Press, 2006.)

Lung cancer

There are two main types of lung cancer: the commonest is called non-small cell lung cancer, which accounts for about four out of five cases of the disease; the other is small cell lung cancer which makes up the other one in five cases.

If possible, the first line treatment for a non-small cell lung cancer is surgery to remove the growth. But this involves taking away quite a lot of lung tissue, and as these tumours are almost always due to smoking, people often have quite severe lung damage already from conditions like bronchitis and emphysema, so to do an operation might be dangerous. Therefore, radiotherapy is often advised as a safer alternative to surgery.

For small cell lung cancer the first line of treatment is chemotherapy, but radiotherapy may sometimes be given at the end of the drug treatment to maximize the benefit.

As with breast cancer, radiotherapy is a very effective form of symptom control, or palliation, for people with advanced lung cancer, and just one or two treatments will ease symptoms like breathlessness, cough, chest pain and coughing up of blood (haemoptysis) for most of them.

Prostate cancer

For early prostate cancer, when the growth is still confined to the prostate gland, the active treatment options are surgery, a radical prostatectomy, or radiotherapy, which may involve either external beam therapy or brachytherapy. For some older men, in whom the condition is likely to be very slow growing and relatively trouble free, it may be safe simply to keep treatment in reserve and only give it if troublesome symptoms develop (this is called watchful waiting, or active surveillance). The chances of a cure are equally good with either surgery or radiotherapy, and this is one situation where the choice of treatment really should be down to individual patients, once they have been fully informed of the pros and cons of the two types of therapy.

For slightly more advanced prostate cancers, when the growth has broken through the wall of the prostate gland into the surrounding tissue, but has not obviously spread elsewhere, radiotherapy is a very effective treatment and is usually combined with hormone drugs. At this stage, which is called locally prostate cancer, surgery is not helpful, and neither is brachytherapy, so the radiotherapy relies on external beam treatment.

Once again, in advanced prostate cancer, where spread of the tumour to the bones is a big problem, radiotherapy can do a lot to ease unpleasant bone pain, so it has a major role in the palliative care of men with metastatic, or secondary, prostate cancer.

Bowel cancer

Bowel cancers may develop in either the colon or the rectum. Radiotherapy is very rarely used for colonic cancer because this part of the bowel is close to organs like the small intestine and the kidneys, which are very sensitive to radiation and could be easily damaged by treatment. The rectum lies deep down in the pelvis and radiotherapy to this area is much safer. Many clinical trials have shown that combining radiotherapy with surgery, either pre-operatively to shrink the tumour, or after surgery, as post-operative adjuvant therapy, greatly reduces the risk of a local recurrence of the cancer in the pelvis. For slightly more advanced rectal cancers that have begun to invade the surrounding pelvic tissues, giving radiotherapy combined with chemotherapy before surgery is a fairly recent development in treatment which is helping to make many of these cancers, that would previously have been incurable, suitable for surgery and a possible permanent cure.

When bowel cancers spread they most often go to the liver, and chemotherapy is the best approach to help control liver secondaries (these days it may sometimes be combined with surgery to remove parts of the liver that have been affected). Occasionally bowel cancers may spread to the bone, and radiotherapy can help ease the pain that this might cause, but overall radiation does not play a big part in the palliation of these cancers.

4

How does radiotherapy work?

For many people radiotherapy is a very mysterious treatment. You can't feel it or see it: an invisible form of energy is somehow being used to treat you. But that energy has to be handled with great care and precision because, while it can have amazing healing power, it may also cause damage and side effects. These days radiotherapy is almost only used to treat cancer, and to understand how it works we need to understand a bit about what a cancer is.

What is a cancer?

We all begin our lives as a single cell fertilized in our mother's womb. That cell then divides to form two cells, those two cells divide to make four, and this process of cell division continues throughout pregnancy and on through infancy, childhood and adolescence to produce the countless billions of cells that make up our adult selves. Even in adulthood the process of cell growth continues, because cells are constantly wearing out and dying off and need to be replaced. For example, the bone marrow, which produces the red cells, white cells and platelets that make up our blood, makes many millions of new cells every day to replace those that have worn out. Similarly, the cells that line parts of our digestive system are replaced every 24–48 hours.

Throughout our lives, these processes of cell division and growth are very precisely controlled so that we make exactly the number of new cells that our bodies need – no more, no less. A cancer develops when the cells in a particular organ escape from these controls and begin to reproduce and grow in a haphazard way, producing more cells than they should. Over time, these cells build up to form a tumour, or growth. If this is not treated, then the growth will begin to invade and destroy the tissue surrounding it. It may also send off seedlings – tiny clumps of cells – that spread to form secondary growths in other parts of the body. These seedlings may be carried either in the bloodstream or through the lymph vessels – the network of thread-like channels that drain fluid from the tissues into the lymph glands (lymph nodes).

Tumours can be divided into two main types: benign and malignant. Benign tumours may grow to a large size, but they do not actually invade and destroy the tissue surrounding them, and they do not spread to other parts of the body. Malignant tumours are able both to invade and destroy nearby tissue, and to form secondary growths. The word 'cancer' only applies to these growths; a benign tumour is not a cancer, but a malignant tumour is. Most cancers start as a single growth in one part of the body; this is called the primary cancer. As it continues to grow, the primary cancer may, or may not, produce secondary cancers elsewhere. Another name for these secondary cancers is metastases. When a doctor or nurse talks about metastatic cancer, they mean a cancer that has already spread to other parts of the body.

How does radiotherapy work?

The process of cell division is controlled by the nucleus, the command centre that lies at the heart of all our cells. Within the nucleus are the genes which control all the cell's activities, including cell division. The genes are made up of a complex protein called DNA.

Radiotherapy relies on the use of ionizing radiations (see Introduction). These are very high-energy forms of radiation, and when a cell receives a dose of ionizing radiation chemicals called free radicals are produced. These free radicals damage the DNA. In addition, the ionizing radiation itself also directly damages DNA. About two-thirds of the effect of radiotherapy on cells is due to free radical formation, and about one-third due to the direct damage of the ionizing radiation. If this damage to the DNA is not repaired, then the cell will not be able to divide, and will eventually die. In this way radiotherapy interferes with cell division, stopping cells from multiplying and causing them to die off.

High-dose, curative radiotherapy

Radiotherapy cannot tell the difference between normal, healthy cells and cancer cells. So when a dose of radiation is given, both normal cells and cancer cells will be damaged. How then can radiotherapy kill off cancers without killing off large numbers of healthy cells, causing severe, or even life-threatening, side effects? The answer lies in a vital difference between cancer cells and normal cells: the difference in their ability to repair injury.

With the typical doses of radiation used in modern-day treatment there will be some damage to the DNA of normal cells. But those cells will be able to repair that damage, and be as good as new, within about four to six hours of the radiation. So in less than eight hours they will have recovered completely. Because they are abnormal, cancer cells are much worse at being able to repair themselves; they can only make good the damage to their DNA caused by the radiation over a period of days or weeks, and they take far longer to recover than normal cells. This means that if you give another dose of radiation 24 hours after the first, then the normal cells will have made good the damage of the day before, but the cancer cells will still be trying to recover. The second dose of radiation will damage the normal cells again, but they will rapidly repair the injury and bounce back. The cancer cells will, however, be further damaged and more critically injured. If this pattern is continued for several weeks, then eventually all the cancer cells will be killed off but the normal cells, although they will have been temporarily injured, will have recovered completely.

So by splitting up treatment into a series of small doses, or fractions, of radiation, it is possible to maximize the damage to the cancer and minimize the damage to normal tissues. This is why, when it is used to try and cure a cancer, radiotherapy is almost always given as a course of treatment over a period of several weeks.

Each of us is a unique individual, and in the same way every cancer is different. This means that although fractionation, splitting a course of radiotherapy into lots of relatively small doses, is the theory that explains why treatment works, it does not guarantee the outcome of treatment. Some cancers will be more resistant than others to the effects of radiation, and some normal tissues will be more sensitive than others to the damage caused by the radiotherapy. So, although many cancers are cured by radiotherapy, there will still be some times when the treatment fails. Similarly, although side effects can usually be kept to a minimum, there will be times when they are more severe and troublesome than expected.

Lower-dose, palliative radiotherapy

As I have said, when used to help cure a cancer, radiotherapy is almost always given as a fractionated course of a number of treatments over several weeks. But very often radiotherapy is given to ease the symptoms of more advanced cancers, rather than in the hope of achieving a cure. This type of treatment, often called palliative radiotherapy, usually involves much lower doses of radiation, and often a single treatment, rather than a course of treatment, is very effective.

Many cancer-related symptoms, such as pain from secondary cancers in the bone (bone metastases), breathlessness from advanced lung cancer, or headache from secondary cancers in the brain (brain metastases), can be eased by a single radiotherapy treatment. Why these low-dose treatments are so effective is a mystery. Radiobiology, the science behind radiotherapy, is at a loss to explain it. But radiotherapy has always been a treatment based on experience as much as science and very often doctors have found ways of using the treatment that are effective, but that scientists have taken a long time to be able to explain.

Oxygen

For radiotherapy to be effective, there must be a good supply of oxygen in the blood. If there isn't enough oxygen in the tissues then the free radicals, the chemicals that cause the effects of the radiation on the DNA in the cells, cannot be produced, so the treatment won't work.

Most of the oxygen in our blood is carried by haemoglobin in the red blood cells. When someone is anaemic it means that there haemoglobin level is low, and this means that there is less oxygen in their blood, which leads to symptoms like tiredness and breathlessness. So if you are anaemic, radiotherapy is less likely to be effective than if your haemoglobin level is normal. Anaemia is quite a common problem for people who have cancer, so if your doctors suspect that you might be anaemic they will do a routine blood test before you start your radiotherapy to check on your haemoglobin level. If the test shows that you are anaemic then they will probably suggest that you have a blood transfusion before starting your course of treatment. This will usually involve a single visit for a few hours as a day-patient and very rarely causes any side effects. It will almost instantly improve your haemoglobin level, and probably make you feel better, with less tiredness and more energy.

5

Dose and treatment scheduling

In its early days, radiotherapy developed more as an art than a science. Doctors really did not understand how or why the radiation was working, they simply looked at what was happening to their patients and used their personal judgement and experience to decide how best to give the treatment. So, many of the foundations of modern-day radiotherapy were laid down on the basis of this trial-and-error, empirical approach.

The early radiotherapists were also limited by the equipment they had available for giving radiotherapy. The first, primitive treatment sets could only deliver low doses of radiation over quite long periods of time. This meant that in order to get a dose that was going to be effective patients had to have a series of treatments over a period of time, with each treatment often lasting an hour or more. Purely by chance, this pattern of dividing up the treatment into a number of visits over a period of days or weeks happens to be the best way of giving higher doses of radiation.

When radiotherapy machines became more efficient, and it was possible to give large doses in a matter of minutes rather than hours or days, doctors found that, with the exception of small skin cancers, giving a single high-dose treatment for cancer was ineffective and often caused severe and unacceptable side effects. So the practice of giving high doses of radiation as a course of treatment, split up into a number of episodes, or fractions, continued and evolved.

Nowadays a single radiotherapy treatment is still often used to treat skin cancer, and relatively low-dose single treatments are also effective to help ease some symptoms related to cancer (like bone pain); but nearly all treatments that are aimed at curing a cancer involve higher doses and a course of treatment, with a variable number of fractions, or visits, over a variable length of time.

Measuring the dose of radiotherapy

For many years the unit used to measure a radiation dose was called the rad. So someone having treatment would have a prescription made out by their specialist stating how many rads of radiation they should get at each visit for their radiotherapy. In 1975 a new unit, called the Gray, was introduced to replace the rad. The Gray was largely a European idea, and there are still some countries around the world that have not taken it up and continue to use the rad as their standard measure for radiation dose. However, it is the unit that is used in the UK, and is usually abbreviated to Gy. One Gray is the same as 100 rads, so some people use yet another unit, the centi-Gray (cGy for short), which is one hundredth of a Gray, because this is the same as the old rad. The Gray is named after Louis Harold Gray (1905–65), a British physicist who studied the effects of ionizing radiation on living tissue, and pioneered the science of radiobiology.

The biological effects of radiation: treatment schedules

What radiotherapy actually does to the tissues that are irradiated, the biological effect of the radiation, depends on the dose that is given: the higher the dose, the greater the effect. But it also depends on at least two other very important things: the number of individual treatments, or fractions, that are used to give that dose, and the number of days or weeks over which those fractions are scheduled. So, for example, a dose of 60 Gray (60Gy) is often given to cure cancer. If that dose of 60Gy were given in a single fraction, at a single treatment session, it would cause severe, permanent damage to the tissues that were irradiated, and might even be fatal. But splitting that same total dose into 30 fractions, with a dose of 2Gy given at each visit, for 5 days a week over 6 weeks, is a safe and effective treatment that has been widely used for many decades.

These days, in most branches of medicine, doctors look at the results of clinical trials to guide their decisions about treatment. But clinical trials have only been around for the last 30 years or so, and before that time different doctors, in different places around the world, had worked out different ways of giving effective radiotherapy for cancer treatment. Because the biological effect of that radiation treatment depends not only on the total dose given, but also the number of fractions used, and the overall time taken, this means that a variety of different treatment schedules produce a similar effect. So, for example, a total dose of 60Gy, given in 30 treatments of 2Gy each, 5 days a week for 6 weeks, has a very similar effect to a dose of 50Gy, given in 20 treatments of 2.5Gy each, for 5 days a week over 4 weeks. So, different hospitals, in different parts of the country, and different parts of the world, have developed different patterns of dose, fractionation and scheduling for their radiotherapy treatments.

In recent years quite a few clinical trials have been done to compare these different recipes for treatment, and by and large they have shown that the various schedules are similar in both their effectiveness as a treatment and their risk of any side effects. This means that if someone living in Manchester with, say, a bladder cancer finds that they are having a different dose and schedule of radiotherapy from a friend who lives in Southampton, it does not mean that one treatment is right and the other is wrong; it just means that there are two different ways of getting the same end result. Similarly, a woman living in one part of the country may find that her course of radiotherapy after surgery for a breast cancer is given as 15 treatments, Monday to Friday over 3 weeks, with a total dose of 40Gy; whereas another woman, in another part of the country might have her treatment given as 25 fractions, Monday to Friday over 5 weeks, with a total dose of 50Gy. The pattern of treatment, and the overall dose of radiation used, is very different, but clinical trials have shown that both schedules are equally effective, and carry a similar, small risk of side effects.

Sensitivity of different cancers to radiation

An important point to mention is that as well as different treatment schedules being used to treat the same type of cancer, different types of cancer will need different doses of radiation. There is no single dose and schedule of radiotherapy that can be used to treat all cancers. Some cancers are much more sensitive to radiotherapy than others, and so need lower doses, while others are much more resistant to treatment and need far higher doses. So someone who is having radiotherapy for, say, a lymphoma, which is a type of cancer which is very sensitive to radiotherapy, would have a very different pattern of treatment to someone who has a prostate cancer, which will need a much higher dose of radiation in order to get a cure.

Missing treatments

If you are having a course of radiotherapy that lasts for four or five weeks, with treatment every Monday to Friday, there may well be times when you are feeling tired or under the weather and would like to miss an occasional day. Does this matter? Unfortunately the answer to this is generally 'Yes'. If you miss a single day during treatment this may not matter too much but missing more might reduce the effectiveness of your treatment.

A lot of research has been done on this subject and continuity of treatment is more important in some situations than others. If you are having curative, high-dose radiotherapy for a cancer of the mouth or throat, a cancer of the cervix (the neck of the womb) or a lung cancer then it is very important not to miss treatments. If you are having curative treatment for a cancer of your gullet (oesophagus), or a cancer of your vagina then gaps in treatment should be avoided. For other cancers where you are having curative radiotherapy it is not so critical but it is still best not to miss a treatment if possible. If you are having the radiotherapy to ease symptoms, rather than for a cure (palliative treatment), then missing occasional visits is less important.

If an interruption to your treatment is unavoidable, for whatever reasons, then your clinical oncologist will try and adjust the dose and schedule of your remaining course to compensate. This may mean adding on the days you have missed at the end of your course, or increasing the overall number of treatments, or increasing the dose of radiation that is given at each of your remaining treatments.

When your treatment is first being planned, if you know of any reason why you might have to miss one or more treatments during your course (for example, a holiday you have booked, or a family wedding), do let your oncologist know so that they can allow for this in scheduling your treatment, or arrange a later date for you to start so that there won't be any gaps in your course.

Phased treatment and boost doses

When it is being used as part of the treatment to try and cure a cancer, radiotherapy may be given in phases or stages. To begin with, quite a large area of tissue is treated to a relatively low dose, and then a further course of treatment is concentrated on a smaller field, within this area, to complete the treatment. The idea behind this is that microscopic traces of cancer spreading out as tiny threads from a primary tumour are likely to be more sensitive to radiation than the main, solid mass of the tumour. So a lower dose can be given covering the tumour and its surroundings, in the hope of killing off those microscopic threads, and then the higher dose that follows is focused on the primary tumour. This also helps keep side effects as low as possible by reducing the amount of tissue that gets a high dose of radiation. For example, when a cancer of the rectum is being treated there may be a first phase of treatment that covers the whole of the pelvis, and then a second phase that cones down just to treat that part of the lower bowel where the cancer is.

A variation to this approach is to treat the particular organ where the primary cancer is, or where it has been removed from by surgery, to a reasonably high dose, and then give a short further course of radiotherapy just to that part of the organ where the tumour is, or was. This is called giving a boost treatment. It is most often done for women who have had a lumpectomy for breast cancer: to begin with they have a course of radiation covering the whole of their remaining breast, and then a short boost course of radiation gives a top-up dose just to that part of the breast where the cancer was.

6

People you will meet

For most people radiotherapy will come a little way along their cancer journey. The first steps will usually be a visit to your GP, who will then refer you on to a specialist surgeon or physician at your local hospital. These specialists will do the tests needed to make a diagnosis, to confirm whether or not you have cancer, and if so what type of cancer you have. They will also do tests to see how big your cancer is, and whether it has spread to nearby lymph nodes, or to other parts of the body (doctors call this staging a cancer, working out what stage it has reached in its growth). Very often, especially if your hospital consultant is a surgeon, he or she will also carry out the first part of your treatment, with an operation to take away your cancer.

Once your doctors know what type of cancer you have, and what stage it has reached, they will meet together as a multi-disciplinary team to decide on how best it should be treated. This multi-disciplinary team will include specialist surgeons or physicians, specialist nurses, and doctors trained to give chemotherapy and radiotherapy. There will also be doctors who are experts at reading X-rays and scans (radiologists), and pathologists, who look at cancer under the microscope to tell exactly what type it is. If the multi-disciplinary team (often called an MDT) decides that you need radiotherapy then they will arrange an appointment for you in your nearest department, and you will then meet the various members of the team who will do your treatment.

Clinical oncologist

The consultant, or specialist, who will be in charge of your radiotherapy is called a clinical oncologist. The word oncologist means a cancer specialist, and there are many different types of oncologist. Surgeons who work mainly with cancer patients will often add the word oncologist to their particular area of interest, so a gynaecological oncologist is a surgeon who specializes in cancers of the womb, cervix and ovary, and a urological oncologist is a surgeon who specializes in cancers of the kidney, bladder and prostate gland.

A clinical oncologist is a doctor who has been trained to treat people using radiotherapy or chemotherapy. Until the mid-1990s these doctors were usually called radiotherapists, but because of their increasing involvement with chemotherapy as well as radiation the name of their specialty was changed. The UK is a little unusual in that in most countries doctors who give radiotherapy are not qualified to give chemotherapy, and specialize exclusively in radiation treatment. They are usually known as radiation oncologists. Doctors who specialize in chemotherapy are called medical oncologists. We have medical oncologists in Britain who are experts in the drug treatment of cancer, but are not qualified to give radiotherapy. So if you live in the UK and are going to have radiotherapy, the consultant in charge of your treatment will be a clinical oncologist. If you are going to have chemotherapy or other drugs to treat your cancer, then you may be under the care of either a clinical oncologist or a medical oncologist.

Sometimes people talk about doctors who specialize in radiotherapy as radiologists. This is incorrect: radiologists are doctors who use X-rays and scans to diagnose cancer and other illnesses, but they are not involved in its treatment. So if you have a CT scan as part of the tests to work out the stage of your cancer, this will be organized by a radiologist, but if you then need treatment with radiotherapy this will be organized by a clinical oncologist.

Most consultant clinical oncologists will have more junior doctors working with them, who are training to become specialists in clinical oncology. These doctors are called specialist registrars, or SpRs for short. The key decisions about your treatment will usually be taken by your consultant but their SpR may see you for check-ups on your progress during and after your course of radiation.

Therapy radiographers, radiotherapists

Your consultant clinical oncologist will plan and supervise your radiotherapy treatment and will be in charge of your care during this time, and may continue to look after you for months or years afterwards. But they will not actually give you your treatment. The people who you will see each time when you come for treatment, and who will look after you on a day-to-day basis during your course of radiation, are called therapy radiographers. At least, that is what they used to be called. In some hospitals in recent years they have taken on the name of 'radiotherapists' (this can be confusing because, as we have seen, clinical oncologists used to be known as radiotherapists until a decade or so ago).

Therapy radiographers, or radiotherapists, are not doctors or nurses, but are skilled clinical staff who have been trained to operate the different types of radiotherapy machine used for cancer treatment, and to look after you while you have treatment: giving advice on possible side effects, checking for any signs of these side effects and helping you to cope with them. They will also be closely involved in the preparation and planning of your course of radio-therapy, before your treatment begins. In some countries therapy radiographers are called radiation technicians.

If your treatment is being given on a linear accelerator (see page 13) then there will usually be three or four therapy radiographers in the team operating that machine. They will make you feel welcome when you come for your treatment, answer your questions and explain what is going to happen. They will do their best to make the whole experience of radiotherapy as pleasant and comfortable as possible.

Mould-room technicians

For some types of radiotherapy special devices have to be made for individual patients. The commonest of these are the masks which people with some cancers of the head or neck wear when they are lying on the treatment couch, during their irradiation (see page 48).

These various items are made in the mould room in the radio-therapy department, and so the people who make them are known as mould-room technicians. You will only see these members of the team if you need a mask or other device made specially for you.

Medical physicists

You probably won't meet a member of the medical physics team while you are having your treatment, but they have a number of vital roles behind the scenes. They are involved in the installation and maintenance of all radiotherapy equipment. They also carry out regular checks to ensure it is safe and accurate.

Medical physicists are also involved in the planning of more complex treatments: taking all the measurements that have been made on patients, and information from scans and X-rays, and entering these on to computers. They then work with your consultant clinical oncologist to produce the plans and prescriptions which the therapy radiographers will use to deliver your treatment.

Nurses

There will be nurses helping your consultant in the outpatient clinic where you are first seen to discuss your cancer and the treatment that you need, and they will also be there in those clinics when you are being followed up after your course of radiotherapy is complete. But, while you are actually having your radiation treatment you probably won't see a nurse unless you need special care, such as having regular dressings for a wound.

Other members of the team

The person who first arranges your appointment is likely to be your clinical oncologist's secretary. They may well phone you to confirm the date and time of your visit, and will usually be the person to contact if you have any queries or problems in between your routine appointment times. If you need help with transport to get to the hospital, then your consultant's secretary will often be the person to arrange this for you.

When you come to the radiotherapy department, the first person you will meet is the receptionist. She or he will do their best to make you welcome, and show you where to go and what to do next. They will start by checking your name, and probably also your date of birth, postcode and the name of your GP – all this may sound a bit formal, but it is done to make sure that they are dealing with the right person and have the right set of hospital notes to go with them, so that no mistakes are made.

If you need a blood test during your treatment then most radiotherapy departments will have a phlebotomist available. This is someone who is specially trained to take blood tests. Often they will also be able to process samples for routine blood counts (checking on whether or not you are anaemic, and how many white blood cells and platelets you have), getting these results through in just a matter of a few minutes, while you wait for them.

If you have problems with mobility then there will also be a team of porters who can help you with wheelchairs, or if necessary a stretcher, to get you from place to place in the hospital. They will also be able to collect medicines from the pharmacy for you, or run other necessary errands.

7

Radiotherapy planning

Once you have met your clinical oncologist and agreed that you need radiotherapy, he or she will explain the details of the treatment, outlining the length of your course of radiation, the number of visits you will have to make and possible side effects you might have. You will have a chance to ask questions, and then, when you are completely satisfied, you will be asked to sign a consent form, confirming that you agree to have the treatment that has been described to you.

Before you start your treatment the next stage will be a period of preparation, or pre-treatment planning. Depending on a number of things, such as where your cancer is, the type of cancer you have, and whether you are having treatment in the hope of getting a cure or simply to ease troublesome symptoms (palliative treatment), this may be very quick and simple, taking only a few minutes, or it may be a complex technical process taking several weeks. However it is done, the aim of pre-treatment planning is always the same: to make sure the radiotherapy is accurately targeted on your cancer, covering all the tumour tissue that needs to be treated, while at the same time trying to keep the amount of surrounding normal tissue that is irradiated to an absolute minimum, so that the risk of side effects is kept as low as possible.

Simple pre-treatment planning

The commonest type of skin cancer is called a basal cell carcinoma, or rodent ulcer. These usually appear as a small spot on the face, usually in older people, which does not heal and grows very slowly over months or even years. Because they are on the face, and clearly visible, they are normally diagnosed when they are still quite small. At this stage these cancers can be cured with a single radiotherapy treatment. The 'planning' for this treatment could not be simpler:

the clinical oncologist just draws a line on your skin, around the cancerous spot, with a margin of about half a centimetre of normal skin, to make sure the growth is fully covered, and that is the area that your therapy radiographers will treat.

With some other conditions where the site of the problem is obvious the planning may be equally easy. For example, when irradiating a swollen mass of cancerous lymph nodes in the groin or the neck, or a painful, tender spot in one of the bones where there is a secondary cancer, it may be possible for your clinical oncologist just to draw on your skin to show the place that needs to be treated.

More complex planning

Most radiotherapy treatments will need more preparation in order to get the best results. The precise details of how this is done will vary from hospital to hospital, but the broad principles are very similar.

The first stage in the process is usually a visit to the simulator. The simulator is a machine that takes X-ray pictures or CT scans of the part of your body that is going to be treated. CT scans are increasingly taking over from X-rays in the planning process as they give more detailed and accurate information about the size and position of a cancer. Incidentally, you may have heard of MRI scans (magnetic resonance imaging scans). These are often used to help diagnose cancers (and, of course, many other conditions) and sometimes give more information than CT scans, but for technical reasons CT scans give more accurate images for radiotherapy planning.

The simulator is run by therapy radiographers and they will explain what is going to happen to you and answer any questions you have. They will then take the necessary scans, or X-rays, and may also take a number of measurements from you. All this information will then be sent to computers in the treatment planning department. Usually you don't need any special preparation beforehand, and you can eat and drink normally on the day of your scan. The scanner is shaped like a ring doughnut, and you lie on a couch which passes through the hole in the middle of the doughnut. The radiographers will position you so that the bit of your body that needs to be treated is lying in that hole, surrounded by the scanner. As only part of your body is in the scanner, and there is quite a bit of space between you and the machine, you shouldn't feel too enclosed or claustrophobic. It usually takes about 10 to 15 minutes to take the scan pictures. This process is absolutely painless, but because it involves radiation you will be in the room by yourself during this time, although the radiographers will be watching you, either through a special window or by CCTV. For some scans you may need to have contrast material to show up certain organs or tissues more clearly. This may either be given as a drink or by an injection into a vein in your arm. You shouldn't have any after effects from the scan and so it is perfectly all right for you to drive yourself to and from hospital for this visit if you would like to.

Once the therapy radiographers are sure they have all the information necessary for planning your treatment they will usually need to make a mark on your skin which will act as a reference point for positioning everything accurately during your actual treatment. Because this mark is very important, and it is essential that it is in the right place throughout your treatment, it is normally made as a small tattoo. This is done by putting a drop of indelible black ink on your skin, and pricking or scratching it once or twice with a sterile needle. This leaves a small dot, about the size of a pinhead. This is a permanent mark, which means you can wash and shower throughout your treatment without the risk of it disappearing. It does, however, mean that it will be there always, but as it is very small most people don't find it a cosmetic problem; if it is in a visible area, and you are worried about it, it can always be covered by a tiny dab of make-up.

If you are really worried about having a tattoo, and really do not want it, then the reference point can be marked with a cross drawn in ink on the skin, which is then covered with sticky tape so that it does not rub off. The therapy radiographers will then refresh the mark each time you come for treatment. But there is the risk of the mark rubbing off or slightly changing position during your course of treatment, so this is a second-best approach compared to having a tattoo.

At the end of your visit to the simulator, the radiographers will probably arrange the date and time for your first treatment, and give you information leaflets and answer any other questions you have thought of about what is going to happen. All in all your visit should last somewhere between 30 and 90 minutes.

Behind the scenes

If your simulator visit involved taking a few X-rays, rather than scans, then it may be that your clinical oncologist will look at these more or less immediately and use them to prescribe your treatment, so that your radiotherapy starts within a day or two, or possibly even the same day. Most situations, however, will need the more detailed information that comes from scans in order to plan your treatment accurately. The scans from the simulator are processed by special computer programmes which produce pictures showing exactly where your cancer is, and how big it is. Your clinical oncologist will look at these pictures and use them to decide how much tissue needs to be irradiated, drawing on the computer screen to show the precise area that will get the dose of radiation he or she has prescribed for you.

Once this has been done, a team of specially trained medical physicists will use these measurements to work out the number of fields of radiation you will need (see page 15), the size of the radiation beam for each of these fields, and their exact position. They will also make sure that this treatment set-up will give the prescribed dose of radiation to your cancer, while keeping the dose to nearby normal tissues as low as possible, to keep the risk of side effects as low as possible.

The end result of this process will be a detailed treatment plan, which shows where your cancer is, the position of the radiation beams, and pattern of the radiation dose (given in dose levels, rather like the contours on a map). This will also include all the information that your therapy radiographers need to make sure that you and your radiotherapy machine are in precisely the correct positions for each part of your treatment (see Figure 4). You are not actually involved in any of this process, which all goes on behind the scenes. Timings vary, but depending on how complicated your

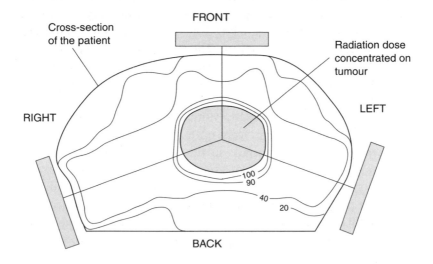

Figure 4 A typical radiotherapy treatment plan for high-dose curative treatment, showing the use of three radiation beams to treat a tumour near the centre of the body

treatment is it may take a couple of weeks to complete this stage of the planning process.

Once your treatment plan has been prepared, you may be asked to come back for another visit to the simulator to check the measurements and scan images against the treatment plan to make sure that it is accurate before you actually start your treatment.

Immobilization, positioning

The great majority of radiotherapy treatments are given on linear accelerators. This means that you will lie on a couch beside the machine, which treats you with a beam of high-energy X-rays. The likelihood is that at each visit the machine will treat you from several different positions. Usually this means that you lie still and the machine will rotate round you each time the position changes, so it's the machine which moves and not you.

To get the best results from treatment it is very important that you are in exactly the right position, and exactly the same position for each of your treatments. Often this can be done simply by your therapy radiographers getting you to lie in a certain way, and lining up the measurements they have from your treatment plan using your tattoo as a reference point. There will also be laser lights at fixed positions in the treatment room shining very accurate beams on the treatment couch, which can also be used to set your position accurately.

One thing you will probably notice is that the couch you are lying on during treatment feels quite hard. This is because it is designed to give a firm surface so that your weight doesn't make it sag or adjust to the shape of your body, which could alter your position slightly during treatment. If you find the couch and your treatment position very uncomfortable your therapy radiographers will usually be able to use pillows or foam cushions to make things easier for you, without changing the position of that bit of you that is being treated.

Sometimes, however, other things are needed to ensure you are correctly positioned. These include:

- *Masks/shells*. These are often used for people who have cancers of the mouth, throat or brain. These are frequently small cancers so targeting the radiation accurately is crucial. The mask is made specially for you so it fits exactly. It has holes cut in it for your eyes, mouth and nose, so you can see and breathe normally. You wear the mask when you are lying on the linear accelerator couch. The mask can be fixed to the couch so it makes sure that you are in the right position, and that you do not move your head during the treatment. This may all sound a little bit frightening but many people become quite attached to their masks and often like to keep them as souvenirs of their treatment! If you do have a mask, then this will mean having to come for one or two visits to another part of the radiotherapy department, called the mould room, where they will prepare your treatment shell. The mask may be made of either clear Perspex or plastic mesh. If you are having a Perspex mask then the first stage of preparation is to make a plaster cast of your face or head. This is done by putting plaster of Paris bandages over your face, leaving space for your mouth and eyes. The bandages will feel warm and wet but dry out in a matter of a few minutes. They are then taken off and will have formed a shell exactly reproducing the contours of your face. This is then used as a mould to make a plaster cast, which in turn is used to act as the template for making the Perspex mask. If plastic mesh is being used, a sheet mesh is gently heated in a water bath and the soft, warm plastic is then moulded over your face; it feels rather like a warm damp towel. As the sheet stretches over your skin tiny gaps appear in the mesh, so it is easy for you to breathe through it. The mesh will dry and harden in a few minutes making a lightweight shell that is then just lifted off. Holes will then be cut in the newly formed mask for your mouth, nostrils and eyes. Having the preparation for your shell is quite painless and takes about 30 minutes.

- *Foot rests.* Moving to the other end of the body, if you are having treatment to your pelvis, for example for a prostate cancer or a rectal cancer, then your therapy radiographers may use a plastic, or carbon fibre, foot rest to help keep you in the right position. This is fitted to the couch of the linear accelerator and is contoured so that your feet and ankles lie snugly in it. This means that you are less likely to move your legs, or wriggle or shift slightly during treatment. The foot rests are a standard piece of equipment made to fit all sizes and so are not made individually.

- *Breast board.* This is specifically for people having radiotherapy to their breast or the front of their chest after surgery to remove a breast cancer. It is a special board which fits between the back of your chest and the couch when you are lying under the linear accelerator. It has a side extension for your arm to rest on, and can be raised to tilt you to the right angle for treatment.

- *Belly board.*   This may be used for some treatments to the pelvis or the belly or the spine. The front part of our belly is filled by the small intestine, and this is very sensitive to radiation and easily damaged by higher doses of radiotherapy. The belly board is a plastic moulding that sits on the couch of the linear accelerator and lifts you a few inches above the level of the couch. It has a hole in the middle. This means that if you lie face down on the belly board, in the right position, then your belly will sag through the hole, keeping most of your small intestine in below the level where you are being treated. Even in thin people this is an effective way of keeping the dose of radiotherapy to the small intestine to a minimum. Once again the belly board is a standard piece of equipment and is not made for individual patients.

Shielding blocks and wedges

The metal jaws, or shutters, in the head of the linear accelerator can be adjusted to form a beam of radiation that is anywhere from a centimetre or two across to one of 30 to 40 centimetres. But because of the shape of the jaws these will produce either a square or rectangular beam. Sometimes it is necessary to produce other shapes, either to cover your cancer more accurately or to protect surrounding normal tissues. Shielding blocks and wedges are two ways of doing this.

Shielding blocks are specially shaped metal alloys that are fixed to a sheet of Perspex. This Perspex sheet is then slotted into the head of the linear accelerator in the path of the radiation beam. Where the blocks are in place they will absorb the radiation and stop it reaching you, in the same way that if you stand in the shade you are protected from the rays of the sun. So by using different-sized blocks to produce these shadows the pattern of the beam of radiation when it reaches the surface of your skin can be adjusted to whatever shape is necessary.

The dose of radiation produced by the beam from a linear accelerator is the same across the whole cross-section of the beam. Sometimes, in order to match the contours of your body, it is better if the dose of radiation is less on one side of the beam than the other. This can be achieved by using wedges. These are made of metal alloys and again fit into the head of the linear accelerator. As they are wedge-shaped they have a thinner end and a thicker end. Some of the radiation from the linear accelerator will be absorbed by the metal in the thicker end of the wedge, much less will be absorbed by the thinner end. When the beam reaches your skin, the part of the beam that has passed through the thin end of the wedge will therefore give you a larger dose of radiation than the part of the beam that went through the thicker part of the wedge.

As a patient you will not be directly involved in the making of shielding blocks or the selection of wedges for your treatment. This will all be done behind the scenes as part of the pre-treatment planning process, based on the X-rays, scans and measurements taken when you came for your simulator visit.

With the latest generation of linear accelerators the jaws in the treatment head of the machine are much more sophisticated (see page 55) and can produce the same changes to the beam as metal shielding blocks or wedges, so if you are having your treatment on one of these newer machines these may not be necessary.

Bolus or build-up

As we have seen, the beam of X-rays from a LinAc passes through the skin without irradiating it and only becomes active a centimetre or so below the skin surface. This has the benefit of reducing the risk of skin damage, which is obviously a good thing. Occasionally, however, there is the risk that there might be traces of cancer in the skin overlying a tumour and this means it is important that the skin is treated in order to get rid of those cells. This is done by putting a sheet of special material, called bolus or build-up, over the area of skin that has to be treated. The bolus acts like an extra layer of body tissue which the beam has to pass through, and its thickness is calculated to bring the radiation to the skin surface. There are different types of bolus: plastic pouches filled with oil, or foam plastic sheets, or other materials, but all will form a soft, rubbery, floppy layer that will mould itself to fit exactly to the contours of your skin. So, without the bolus the beam passes through the first centimetre of tissue that it meets and then begins to give up its radiation energy; with the bolus it passes through a centimetre or so of bolus and then begins to give out radiation as soon as it meets the skin.

8

Special types of radiotherapy

Electron beam therapy

A linear accelerator (LinAc) works by producing a high-energy beam of electrons which is fired at a metal target in the head of the treatment machine. The interaction between the electrons and the target produces the beam of X-rays which is then directed to treat the patient. In some LinAcs the target can be moved out of the way so that the electron beam itself is used for the treatment, rather than a beam of X-rays.

Electrons are absorbed in human tissue in a different way to X-rays. The high-energy beam of X-rays from a LinAc usually shoots through the first centimetre or so of tissue it meets before it then begins to give out its radiation. The deeper it penetrates into the tissue, the more the radiation is absorbed and the weaker the beam becomes. So there is a steady fall off in the intensity of the beam the further it penetrates. By contrast, the electron beam starts giving off radiation as soon as it hits the skin, and gives off a fairly constant level of radiation for the next few centimetres of tissue it goes through, and then the radiation level falls off very sharply so that almost no radiation energy passes to deeper levels.

This difference in the distribution of radiation of the two types of beam means that for a few cancers, especially some skin cancers, and certain cancers of the mouth and throat, using the electron beam of a LinAc may give better results than using the normal X-ray beam.

Total-body irradiation (TBI)

Total-body irradiation is a type of radiotherapy given to people who are going to have a bone-marrow transplant as part of their treatment for cancers like leukaemia, lymphoma or myeloma. The aim of treatment is to destroy cancer cells in the bone marrow throughout the body; this also destroys normal bone-marrow cells and so the treatment is followed immediately by the transplant, to replace the normal cells.

Total-body irradiation is given by a LinAc and usually involves treatment twice a day, morning and evening, for between three and eight doses. The whole body is irradiated and although the dose of radiation is quite low, because the treatment is so extensive it can cause quite a lot of side effects, especially the risk of infection. Because of this it does mean that you have to be in hospital while the treatment is given.

Proton therapy

Proton therapy uses a machine called a cyclotron to produce a beam of heavy ionizing particles called protons. The advantage of proton therapy over normal radiotherapy, using the X-ray beam from a LinAc, is that the proton beam can be more precisely targeted on the cancer, with little irradiation of surrounding normal tissue, so there are fewer side effects.

Proton beam therapy has been mainly used to treat three types of cancer: a special type of malignant melanoma occurring in the retina, at the back of the eye (ocular melanomas), and two very rare cancers, chondrosarcomas and chordomas, affecting the tissues in the lower part of the skull and the upper part of the spine.

In the UK the only cyclotrons that are available for treating patients produce relatively low-energy beams, which can only be used for treating ocular melanomas. Higher-energy beams are needed to treat the chordomas and chondrosarcomas of the base of the skull and the spine. A few such machines are available at centres in the USA and some parts of Europe, and the Department of Health will pay for treatment of carefully chosen patients at one of these centres in other countries if this is felt to be the best treatment for them.

Although some doctors are campaigning for high-energy proton beam cyclotrons in Britain, others argue that the development of conformal radiotherapy (see below) means that this is no longer necessary.

Neutron therapy

Cyclotrons can also be used to produce a beam of ionizing particles called neutrons. The advantage of a neutron beam compared to a normal X-ray beam is that neutrons do not need a good supply of oxygen in the cancer tissue for them to be effective. This discovery led to the hope that neutron therapy might be effective in certain types of cancer that were known to have a very poor blood supply, and hence very low oxygen levels. However, a number of clinical trials carried out during the late twentieth century, comparing neutron therapy with conventional X-ray treatment with LinAcs, failed to show convincing benefits and did show quite a lot in the way of side effects, so only a few centres around the world have continued research into this type of radiotherapy.

Conformal radiotherapy and intensity modulated radiotherapy (IMRT)

In the past the metal jaws in the head of LinAcs have been simple structures, able to open or shut to various widths, producing a beam of radiation of uniform intensity, with a square or rectangular cross section. In recent years the technology has improved and now the jaws are made up of a number of layers, or leaves of metal, each of which can be positioned separately. This new type of jaw is known as a multi-leaf collimator (MLC). This new technology means that the beams of radiation from a LinAc can be shaped far more precisely than previously. As a result of this, the treatment can be targeted to match the shape of a cancer more closely than in the past. This is called conformal radiotherapy (because the treatment conforms more closely to the shape of the cancer). Conformal radiotherapy has two possible benefits. First, less normal tissue will be irradiated and so the risk of side effects should be reduced. Second, it may allow an increase in the dose of radiation to the cancer, which might increase the chance of a cure. At present clinical trials are showing that this approach to treatment does seem to reduce side effects; whether it increases cure rates still remains to be seen.

A development of conformal radiotherapy is called intensity modulated radiotherapy (IMRT). This once again uses radiation beams shaped by multi-leaf collimators, but uses more beams than normal, each of which is divided into a number of smaller 'beamlets' of different shapes and sizes. This means that the intensity of the radiation within the beam can be varied, to give a very precise three-dimensional coverage of the tumour. This can be very useful where the cancer lies close to, or wraps around, a particular organ to which the radiation dose needs to be reduced.

The planning of intensity modulated radiotherapy is much more complicated, and the actual treatment time when you are lying on the couch under the LinAc is longer. Also, because of the large number of beams used the amount of normal tissue irradiated is greater than with normal radiotherapy, and this has led to some concerns about possible long-term complications from treatment.

At the moment conformal radiotherapy is still being phased in and is not universally available in the UK. Intensity modulated radiotherapy is only on offer in a few centres in Britain. So far these treatments are still being developed and their benefits remain uncertain. For most types of cancer there is no evidence that they offer more than the more traditional approach to treatment. At the present time the cancers where most research has been done are prostate cancer, some types of lung cancer and some cancers of the head and neck, so if you have one of these tumours you may be offered conformal radiotherapy.

Intra-operative radiotherapy (IORT)

Radiotherapy is often given after surgery has been carried out to remove a primary cancer. The aim of the treatment is to prevent a local recurrence of the cancer, with re-growth of the tumour at the site of the operation. The treatment typically involves a course of radiotherapy given by a LinAc over a period of several weeks. Another way of doing this is to give the radiotherapy as a single dose at the time of the operation; this is known as intra-operative radiotherapy, or IORT.

The potential advantages of intra-operative radiotherapy are that people could be spared several weeks of visits for conventional radiotherapy; the amount of normal tissue that is irradiated would be less than with external radiotherapy, and this might reduce the risk of side effects.

A number of machines have now been developed which can produce beams of X-rays or electrons that give very intensive radiation over a distance of a centimetre or so. These machines are relatively small and can be used in an operating theatre. They have special applicators that can be inserted into the space left in the tissues after a cancer has been removed. The machine will then give an intensive dose of radiation to the walls of that cavity and a margin of tissue of a centimetre or so round about. The treatment lasts up to about 30 minutes.

Intra-operative radiotherapy could be used instead of, or as well as, a course of external radiotherapy from a LinAc. At the present time this is still an experimental form of radiotherapy and is not widely available in Britain. The main interest in its use is as a possible alternative to external radiotherapy for some patients having treatment after surgery for early breast cancer, and a large clinical trial is underway to explore this.

Chemoradiotherapy

Many people having treatment for cancer will have both chemo-therapy and radiotherapy. The two types of treatment are usually given for different reasons. The radiotherapy is focused on the primary tumour, or the site where the tumour has been removed by surgery, and is intended to kill off cancer cells in that area. The chemotherapy passes into the bloodstream and goes to all parts of the body in the hope of killing off any traces of cancer that have spread elsewhere. Usually the chemotherapy will be given first, followed later by the radiotherapy.

In the treatment of some types of cancer the combination of radiotherapy and chemotherapy is used differently. Research has shown that, for a few types of cancer, giving chemotherapy at the same time as radiotherapy can make the primary tumour more sensitive to the radiotherapy and make treatment more effective. The chemotherapy is acting as a radiosensitizer, to increase the chance of curing the primary cancer; it is not being given to re-duce the chance of the spread of the cancer. When radiotherapy and chemotherapy are given at the same time in this way it is called chemoradiotherapy. At present the kinds of cancer where this approach to treatment is most often used is for some rectal cancers (cancers of the lower part of the bowel), some mouth and throat cancers, and cervical cancers (cancers of the neck of the womb). Chemoradiotherapy is usually only given for slightly more advanced primary cancers, where it is suspected that there is some growth of the tumour into the surrounding normal tissues.

Hyperfractionation: CHART

When it is used to help cure a cancer, radiotherapy is typically given on a daily basis for five days a week, Monday to Friday, over a number of weeks. But we have seen that the damage that radiotherapy causes to normal cells is repaired within four to six hours. If the next treatment is delayed until the following day this means there will be a period of about eighteen hours when the normal cells will have recovered, a time during which the cancer cells can also begin to repair the damage done to them. With this in mind, scientists have argued that radiotherapy would be more effective if it was given more frequently, with two or three treatments each day, and no break in treatment at weekends. In theory at least, this would maximize the lethal effect of radiotherapy on cancer cells, while still allowing time for normal tissue recovery.

Giving more than one radiotherapy treatment each day is called hyperfractionation. If there is no weekend break it means that the treatment is being given continuously. With multiple daily treatments and no weekend break, the course of radiation is completed much more quickly; it is therefore an accelerated course. This has led to this type of treatment being called CHART, the initials standing for Continuous, Hyperfractionated, Accelerated, RadioTherapy.

Clinical trials of CHART-like treatment have been carried out mainly in certain types of lung cancer and cancers of the mouth and throat (head and neck cancer). The results suggest that CHART may slightly increase the chance of a cure. While this is good news, actually organizing CHART is very difficult. Operating a radiotherapy department twenty-four hours a day to allow CHART to take place is hugely expensive and complicated, and many patients do not like the idea of having to come for two or three visits every day. Overall, these difficulties probably outweigh the small benefits that the treatment might offer. At the present time a few centres in the UK are continuing research into CHART, but it is not in widespread use.

Radioiodine therapy

This treatment involves swallowing capsules, or a drink, containing radioactive iodine. The iodine goes into the bloodstream and is then concentrated in the thyroid gland, in the front of the neck. The radioiodine then irradiates the gland, killing off the thyroid cells.

Radioiodine treatment is the one common use of radiotherapy for a non-cancerous condition. In the UK about 10,000 people every year have radioiodine as treatment for an overactive thyroid gland (hyperthyroidism, or thyrotoxicosis). Sometimes radioiodine may also be used as part of the treatment of thyroid cancers.

Radioiodine has few side effects, but it does stop the thyroid gland from working. This means that most people who have the treatment will need to take daily tablets of thyroid hormone (thyroxine) for the rest of their lives.

Unlike most other types of radiotherapy, radioiodine treatment does mean that you are radioactive for a few weeks after your treatment. This means that there are a number of dos and don'ts about mixing with other people in the first few weeks after treatment. These restrictions are quite detailed and vary according to the dose you have been given. If your doctors suggest radio-iodine to you they should give you all the detail of what you can and can't do after treatment so that you can make an informed decision about having it.

9
Side effects

The idea of radiation causes all kinds of fears and alarms. The after effects of the atomic bombs on Hiroshima and Nagasaki, the Chernobyl explosion, constant scare stories in the media about the dangers of nuclear power, and countless books and movies where ionizing rays cause terrifying mutations or transformations have all left a widespread anxiety in modern-day society about the hazards of ionizing radiation. A fear which, it must be said, is largely based on ignorance and misunderstanding.

After more than a hundred years of worldwide use in medical treatment radiotherapy has proved itself to be not only effective, but safe. Yes, there may be side effects, but these are well understood, generally predictable, usually short-lasting and seldom severe. Certainly the life-changing mutations, the glowing in the dark or bizarre deformities so beloved of science fiction are just that – fiction. They definitely do not happen after radiotherapy!

Before looking in more detail at the side effects that may occur as a result of radiation treatment it is worth making a few general points.

- The risk of side effects relates mainly to the dose of radiation that is given during a course of treatment: the higher the dose the more likely they are to occur. This also means that many people who only have relatively low doses of radiation during their treatment will have little or nothing in the way of upset.
- The side effects of radiotherapy are mostly localized. This means that they tend to affect only the part of the body that is being treated. This is in contrast to chemotherapy, where drugs circulate in the bloodstream throughout the body and so have a more general effect on well-being. The only common general effect of radiotherapy is tiredness, and we will look at this in a bit more detail shortly before going on to talk about the side

effects that might happen when different parts of the body are treated.

- The side effects of treatment may be either immediate, developing during or shortly after a course of radiotherapy, or they may be long term, appearing months or sometimes years later. These long-term side effects are much less common than the immediate effects, but they can sometimes be permanent.

- The short-term side effects are due to the radiation causing inflammation in the normal tissues that are included in the treatment. Usually this inflammation will settle down and disappear a while after the treatment is over. But sometimes, particularly after higher doses, there may be permanent changes in the blood supply to those tissues, which lead to long-lasting alterations, causing permanent scarring or damage.

- The sensitivity to the effects of radiation of different tissues and organs in the body varies very considerably. For example, quite low doses will inflame and injure the lungs or the kidneys, whereas much higher doses would be needed to cause the same amount of damage to the brain or the bladder. This means that even when the same dose is being given the side effects of treatment will be very different in one part of the body compared to another.

- With modern-day radiotherapy equipment the risk of side effects, and the severity of those side effects when they do occur, is generally far less than was the case twenty or thirty years ago. So if you have friends or relatives who were treated by radio-therapy before about 1980, or if you come across older books or papers on the subject, they may give you a very false impression of the adverse effects of treatment.

- Finally, there is individual variation. Each of us is different, and because of this people having identical treatments will find that they have different side effects, or experience a particular side effect with a greater or lesser degree of upset. For example, one person having radiotherapy to their belly may get some nausea, or even vomiting, while someone else, having just the same dose of radiation for just the same cancer, will have no upset at all. So if you know someone who has had radiotherapy and they had a troublesome side effect it doesn't mean that you will get the same problem.

Tiredness

This is far and away the commonest side effect of radiotherapy. More than seven out of ten people who have a course of radiotherapy lasting more than a week are likely to feel some tiredness. Often the changes are quite slight but sometimes they can be really troublesome and upsetting, seriously interfering with the quality of your life. When these more severe problems occur doctors often call it radiation fatigue: a profound form of tiredness that may not be eased simply by resting.

The main feelings you get with radiation fatigue are physical, with a loss of energy, feeling unable to do anything, and reduced stamina, finding the things you would normally do are either much harder or completely impossible. You feel exhausted, drained, worn out, shattered. A number of other things can go along with this: your sleep may be disturbed – either having difficulty sleeping, or finding you are drowsy and dropping off during the daytime; you may become forgetful or have difficulty in concentrating on things; you may become irritable or tetchy; you may lose interest in things, including food and sex.

Sometimes this fatigue can tip over into clinical depression, which is another, much less common, side effect of the treatment. In this situation you may feel utterly miserable and hopeless, with a complete loss of interest in everything, no motivation to do anything, and a belief that things simply can't and won't get any better.

The tiredness associated with radiotherapy can affect people at all ages, but is more likely in people over 40. Usually it will begin to disappear within a month of finishing your course of treatment, but it may take many more months, or even a year or two, for things to get completely back to normal. Once again, the older you are, the longer the tiredness is likely to last.

The likelihood of troublesome tiredness also varies according to which part of your body is being treated. About four out of five people having radiotherapy to their chest will get radiation fatigue; about two out of every three people having treatment to their belly or pelvis will feel very tired, as will about half of all people having treatment to their head or neck. But people having radiotherapy to an arm or a leg are unlikely to get any tiredness at all.

Sickness: nausea and vomiting

Many people expect that having radiotherapy will make them feel sick. In fact this is quite uncommon. Certainly if you are having radiotherapy to the upper part of your belly, or the middle part of your spine, where the radiation is likely to cover your stomach or large parts of your small intestine, then you may well feel queasy and sick at times, but with most other treatments sickness is unlikely.

The skin

Whenever external beam radiotherapy is given some part of the skin will always be exposed to the radiation. If the treatment is being delivered by a high-energy linear accelerator, as most treatments are these days, then the skin will usually receive only a small dose of radiation, since most of the effects of that treatment occur below skin level in the deeper tissues. But sometimes it may be necessary to include the skin within the area receiving the full dose, in order to completely cover tissues that are at risk. When this happens, skin changes are likely.

Another way in which the skin can be affected is by something called the exit dose of radiation. This can happen with treatment to various parts of the body but perhaps the easiest way to explain it is to think of a cancer in the muscles of the thigh. This might be treated with a single beam of radiotherapy, from a LinAc, directed at the front of the thigh. Because the radiation takes place beneath the surface, the skin on the front of the thigh won't be affected. But even after it has passed through the tissues of the thigh there will still be a lot of energy left in the beam when it passes through the skin at the back of the thigh, and the skin here will get a fair dose of radiation. So although the treatment is being given from the front of the leg, it will be the skin at the back of the leg, where the beam has exited from the tissues, that is actually affected by the radiation.

With small doses of radiotherapy there will be no effect on the skin. As the treatment course progresses, and the cumulative dose of radiation increases, the first change will be some reddening and irritation, or itching, of the skin. For people with brown or black skins, their skin is likely to become darker. For most people this is likely to be the only side effect they will see. Sometimes, however, with higher doses, or for people with more sensitive skins, the itching may turn into soreness, and the reddening progress to some peeling of the skin (a condition that doctors call dry desquamation). In the most severe reaction to treatment the skin becomes blistered and peels, leaving the underlying surface raw, red and weeping with clear fluid (this is called moist desquamation). Moist desquamation is very uncommon and will only affect a tiny minority of people who have radiotherapy.

During a typical course of radiotherapy, where the skin is being irradiated, side effects will usually appear during the second or third week of treatment and gradually build up as the course continues. Once the treatment stops the effects of radiotherapy still carry on in the skin for a while afterwards, so the symptoms may get worse for 10 to 14 days after the end of treatment before things start to improve. Generally speaking, even when moist desquamation (the most severe type of skin damage) is present, once things begin to improve they get better very quickly, with the skin being virtually back to normal within a week or two.

Sometimes during a course of treatment the radiation will stimulate the cells in the skin that contain the pigment melanin (called melanocytes), which gives our skin its colour. This means that during the treatment and for a few weeks afterwards, your skin may go rather darker than normal. This is only a temporary change. Sometimes, with very high-dose treatments, after first stimulating the melanocytes the radiation will go on to permanently damage the cells, and this may mean that the skin in the treated area becomes paler than it was before; this is a permanent change.

Usually there are no long-term side effects from these skin reactions, but occasionally if the skin has been quite severely inflamed then the scar tissue that forms as a result may leave it feeling a little thicker and firmer than normal, although it is unlikely to look any different.Very infrequently, after an intense skin reaction, tiny blood vessels on the surface of the skin may become more prominent, leaving a pattern of tiny red, spidery dots on the skin in the irradiated area, which will be permanent (doctors call these radiation telangiectasia).

The skin also contains the sweat glands and sebaceous glands, which produce oils which help to soften and lubricate the skin. Both these glands will be affected by radiotherapy and lose some of their activity. With higher doses they may stop working permanently. This means that the skin in the irradiated area will no longer sweat (which some people might think is an added benefit of treatment), and the loss of sebaceous glands will mean the skin tends to become drier and less supple.

One special, but common, situation to mention is people who are having treatment for non-melanoma skin cancers (basal cell carcinomas, or rodent ulcers, and squamous cell carcinomas). Most of these are small growths, only a centimetre or two in size at most, and can be treated with a single X-ray exposure, using a superficial radiotherapy machine. This means giving quite a high dose of radiation to the skin, which leads to a fairly uniform pattern of side effects. About a week after the treatment the patch of skin that has been treated will become red, inflamed and itchy. Over the next week or so this reaction will become more intense and the skin may well blister and weep clear fluid, or even bleed a little. At this stage it will look as though the treatment has made things much worse, rather than better, and it is very important to realize that this is just what should be happening; it is not a sign of anything going wrong, or the cancer getting worse. About three to four weeks after treatment the inflammation will begin to settle, the skin will dry and form a crust, like a normal scab after a cut or injury. A week or two later this scab will peel away, leaving new pink skin underneath (with no sign of the original cancer). Over the coming months this new skin will gradually mature to have the same appearance as the normal skin around it. The cosmetic effect after these treatments is usually very good, and it is often very difficult to tell where the treatment was given. Sometimes the irradiated area will stay rather paler than the surrounding skin, and occasionally little spots of radiation telangiectasia will develop in this paler skin.

One uncommon effect on the skin is known as a recall reaction. This can happen when someone who has had radiotherapy months, or even years, previously is given chemotherapy and occasionally the drugs will cause the skin in the area that was treated previously to begin to go red and inflamed, just as though it had been irradiated again. This is usually a short-lived reaction to the drugs, settling in a matter of days, and is not serious.

Hair loss

When they first learn they will need radiotherapy many people worry that they will lose their hair. In fact, because the treatment only affects that part of the body that is being irradiated you will only lose your hair in that area. (This is different to the hair loss that can occur with chemotherapy, where you lose hair every-where.) So if you are having radiotherapy to your head, then you may lose some of your scalp hair; if you are having radiotherapy to the armpit (the axilla), you will lose some of your underarm hair; and if you are having treatment to your pelvis, then you may well lose some of your pubic hair.

The risk of hair loss depends on the dose of radiation given. With low doses there will be no change but with higher doses some hair loss is likely, usually three to four weeks after the treatment starts. Again, depending on the dose, there may be just some thinning of the hair or it may be lost completely. Very often the hair will grow again a few months later, though it may be thinner and finer than before. But with the higher doses used for some curative treatments the hair loss may well be permanent over the particular patch of skin that has been irradiated.

The breast

Giving a course of radiotherapy to the breast after removal of an early breast cancer is probably the most frequent use of radiation treatment to help cure cancer. Every year in the UK alone tens of thousands of women will have this treatment, so it is worth spending a bit of time looking at the possible side effects in some detail. The treatment will include the breast tissue that is left after surgery, and a margin of surrounding normal tissue, as well as a small section of the underlying lung; sometimes the glands under the arm (the axillary lymph nodes) next to the breast will be included in the treatment.

Effects of radiotherapy on the breast

When radiation treatment is given to the breasts after surgery for breast cancer it is important that the skin overlying the breast gets the full dose of radiation, so the changes of pinkness and soreness of the skin described above are very common. One place that is particularly affected is the skin in the fold under the breast, between the breast and the chest.

The breast tissue itself will also become inflamed, and towards the end of the course of treatment the breast may sometimes feel sore and tender and be slightly puffy and swollen, but these changes are usually very short-lived and settle within a week or two of finishing the treatment. In the longer term the radiation will cause fine scar tissue to form (this is called fibrosis) and this will make the breast feel slightly firmer than before. These changes are also likely to make the irradiated breast slightly smaller in size. About half of all women who have this type of radiotherapy will notice some change in the feel and appearance of their treated breast. These changes come on slowly in the months and years after treatment, but generally stabilize after three to five years, with further changes more than five years after radiotherapy being uncommon. Although these changes are more likely with higher doses of radiation there is a lot of individual variation, and so it is difficult to predict in advance what the long-term cosmetic effects of treatment will be for any one person, but, as a general rule, the larger the breasts the more likely it is that there will be both short-term inflammation and discomfort and long-term thickening and shrinkage of the breast tissue. Fewer than one in ten women with small breasts are likely to notice any long-term difference, compared to about four in ten women with large breasts. In women who have had a mastectomy and who then go on to have radiotherapy to the front of their chest (the chest wall), covering the operation scar and the surrounding skin, the side effects they might experience are the same as those described in the section on 'Skin' above.

The underlying lung

Post-operative radiotherapy to the breast or chest wall will always include some of the underlying lung tissue, although careful planning of the treatment keeps this to a minimum. Even so a small number of women who are treated may get some side effects from the lung irradiation. The most common of these is a temporary inflammation called radiation pneumonitis. This develops between one and six months after the end of treatment and causes a dry cough, some shortness of breath and sometimes a slight fever. These symptoms are usually mild and settle down after a few weeks, but occasionally they can be more troublesome. Very rarely the symptoms persist and become permanent, but this is only likely if, for some reason, quite a lot of lung tissue has been included in the treatment. These symptoms are due to scar tissue (fibrosis) form-ing in the part of the lung that has been irradiated. More than eight out of ten women who have breast or chest-wall radiotherapy will develop this fibrosis, although most will never have any symp-toms or problems as a result. However, the fibrosis will show up on any future X-rays of their chest, as a hazy patch, and it is impor-tant to be aware of this and not be worried by it.

The ribs

The ribs supporting the wall of the chest lie between the breast and the lungs and so will be included in the radiation beam. As a result, over a period of years after treatment, the irradiated ribs may become slightly thinner and more brittle, and so are more likely to crack or fracture. Very often if these fractures do occur they are quite painless, but they may be very slow to heal.

The heart

Older reports looking at the results of post-operative radiotherapy in women who had breast cancer raised anxieties about the possible risks of damage to the muscle of the heart from the irradiation. But these studies were looking at the long-term results of old-fashioned ways of giving radiotherapy, and more recent studies, where modern-day types of treatment have been used, show little or no evidence of any risk to the heart. This is because with present-day equipment, and the increased sophistication of pre-treatment planning, the radiation dose to the heart is normally very small indeed.

Lymphoedema

Lymphoedema is a gradual build-up of fluid (lymph) in the arm on the side that has been irradiated. It comes on gradually after the end of treatment, appearing anywhere from one to five years after radiotherapy. Very often the changes are slight, with the arm feeling a bit fuller or heavier, and some mild tightness or stretching of the skin. But sometimes the build-up of fluid can be considerable, leading to very obvious swelling of the arm, which in turn causes pain and stiffness, together with thickening of the skin and underlying tissues (doctors often call this brawny oedema).

The risk of getting lymphoedema, and the severity of the problem, relate mainly to the treatment of the axillary lymph nodes. These nodes form part of the lymphatic system and help drain fluid from the arm through the network of lymph vessels that run throughout the tissues. Both surgery and radiotherapy can damage this drainage system, reducing the flow of lymph and so causing a build-up of fluid in the arm.

Going back twenty years or so, typical treatment for early breast cancer involved surgery to the axilla, removing all the lymph glands (an axillary clearance), followed by high-dose radiotherapy to the area. As a result lymphoedema was a very common complication. These days most women will have either surgery or radiotherapy to their axilla but are unlikely to have both. This has greatly reduced the risk of lymphoedema, but still about one in five to one in ten women will notice some degree of long-term swelling of their arm after either surgery or irradiation. Unfortunately the changes in the tissues under the arm that cause lymphoedema cannot be reversed, so once the condition develops it is permanent. There is no exact way of predicting who will or will not get lymphoedema, but women are more at risk if the lymph glands under their arm contained cancer, or if the surgery there was very extensive, or if a very high dose of radiotherapy was used in their treatment.

The shoulder

Some women do notice stiffness and discomfort in their shoulders, making some arm movements uncomfortable, developing in the years after radiotherapy to their breast or chest wall. This is due to fibrosis developing in the muscles around the shoulder joint and in the joint itself. This problem is more likely if radiotherapy is given to the lymph nodes under the arm, if the person being treated has already got problems with arthritis in their shoulder joint, or if they have lymphoedema of the arm. These symptoms are fairly uncommon and usually mild.

The chest

Radiotherapy to the chest is most often given to treat cancers affecting the lung or the gullet (the oesophagus). Most lung cancers develop in the main airways into the lung (the bronchi) and these lie deep in the centre of your chest (in an area that doctors call the mediastinum). The gullet is a muscular tube that runs through the mediastinum, joining your throat to your stomach. Our lungs lie either side of the mediastinum and so usually they are not affected very much by radiotherapy to the centre of the chest; side effects of breathlessness and cough (as described above) are uncommon. The main side effects are due to irritation of the gullet and this leads to soreness when you swallow, and sometimes pain deep in the chest. If the gullet gets very inflamed then it may be difficult to swallow solid food. This inflammation in the gullet builds up over the first two or three weeks of treatment and will usually settle and disappear within a month or so of completing your radiotherapy.

The central nervous system

The central nervous system is made up of three parts: the brain, the spinal cord and the peripheral nerves. The spinal cord runs from the brain to about two-thirds of the way down the backbone. The peripheral nerves run from the spinal cord to supply the muscles and tissues throughout the body.

The brain

Brain tissue is relatively resistant to radiotherapy which means that side effects usually only appear when high doses of radiation are given. The frontal lobes of the brain (the cerebral hemispheres) are least affected by the effects of radiation, while the tissues of the brain stem (the lowermost part of the back of the brain) are the most sensitive.

The immediate side effects of radiotherapy are due to slight swelling of the brain tissue, caused by inflammation from the treatment. This leads to symptoms like headache, sickness and tiredness. Unless particularly high doses of radiotherapy are being used, these side effects are very unlikely. Long-term side effects of radiotherapy to the brain are due to damage to the blood vessels leading to death of some brain tissue, but once again these changes are very rare unless abnormally high doses of radiation are given.

One change that can occur particularly in children after brain irradiation is called somnolence syndrome. This comes on about four to six weeks after the treatment is over. The child becomes quite sleepy and often complains of feeling sick and unwell. Occasionally other symptoms will appear, including being irritable and miserable, unsteadiness when walking, going off food and running a slight temperature. These symptoms disappear on their own after one to three weeks.

The brain is, of course, housed within the skull, which is covered by the skin of the scalp. This means that radiotherapy to all or part of the brain usually includes some of the hair, and so some hair loss is likely when the brain is irradiated.

The spinal cord

In contrast to the brain, and the peripheral nerves, the spinal cord is quite sensitive to radiation. The only short-term side effect of treatment is a feeling of tingling, or electric shocks, radiating out from the spine and down the limbs when the head is bent forward and the chin tucked onto the chest (which stretches the upper part of the spinal cord). Doctors have called this Lhermitte's sign of electrical paraesthesia. This develops between two and four months after radiotherapy to the spinal cord has been completed. It is often mild, causing little trouble, and probably frequently goes unnoticed. For these reasons nobody is sure just how often it happens.

Usually the temporary changes that cause Lhermitte's sign get better on their own, but occasionally, especially at higher radiation doses, they will gradually get worse and can lead to permanent damage to the spinal cord, which might lead to numbness and tingling and loss of muscle function (paralysis) in some parts of the body.

The peripheral nerves

The peripheral nerves are very resistant to radiotherapy, and even with high doses damage to these nerves from radiation is very rare.

Mouth and throat

A sore mouth

When we look at the inside of our mouths in a mirror we can see that the lining of the cheeks, the gums, the back of the throat and the surface of the tongue look red and moist. This is because they are covered by a thin layer of lining tissue called the oral mucosa. Most of the side effects that occur when radiotherapy is given to cancers in the mouth or throat are due to changes in the mucosa.

The first change is that as the mucosa becomes inflamed by the treatment it changes colour to a deeper, brighter red (doctors call this erythema). With higher doses of treatment the mucosa begins to produce a filmy white coating, made up of a substance called fibrin. To begin with the fibrin appears as white patches, or islands, scattered across the part of the mucosa that is being treated. As the radiotherapy continues these patches merge to form a confluent white film. At higher doses still this film will break down with ulcers forming in the underlying mucosa, and possibly some bleeding from the lining tissues. When this occurs there is a risk of a further complication because the ulcerated mucosa can become infected. As well as leading to an infection in the local tissues there is the risk that this might spread into the bloodstream and lead to a more serious generalized infection, called septicaemia.

These changes in the mucosa are accompanied by increasing soreness and discomfort. By the time the fibrin patches begin to appear the soreness is likely to be sufficient to interfere with normal eating and drinking, and if the inflammation gets worse then these problems will increase.

The severity of inflammation, and of side effects, depends mainly on the dose of radiation being given. Most people having a course of radiotherapy to their mouth or throat will have some symptoms, but only those having high doses are likely to get severe problems with ulceration and the risk of infection. These changes come on gradually during treatment, typically beginning during the second week and gradually increasing as the course continues. Things often continue to get worse for a week or so after the treatment ends, and then steadily drift back to normal over a period of a few weeks.

A dry mouth

Radiotherapy to the mouth or throat will often include some of the salivary glands. These are the glands in and around the tissue of the mouth and throat which make the saliva that keeps our mouths moist.

Higher doses of radiotherapy stop the salivary glands from working properly, and either stop them from making saliva or alter the quality of the saliva, so that it is thick and stringy rather than a clear liquid. This means your mouth and throat become very dry. It also means that it might be more difficult to eat solid food, and that your food will taste different. A lack of saliva also increases the risk of infections in the mouth and gums, and may even make it difficult to talk at times.

With moderate doses of radiation these changes will be temporary and the salivary glands will recover within a few months of completing treatment. But at the higher doses, needed for the cure of some cancers, the changes will unfortunately be permanent.

The teeth

If the area being irradiated includes part of the gums, then care has to be taken over the condition of the teeth. If you have problems with decay or infection then these might be made much worse by radiotherapy. Similarly, if you develop dental problems and need treatment during or shortly after a course of radiation then this might lead to problems.

A stiff jaw

Some radiotherapy treatments to the mouth or throat might include the hinge joint where your jaw meets your skull. This is called the temporomandibular joint, and lies just in front of your ear. Irradiation of this joint can lead to stiffness and limitation of movement, which mean that it is more difficult to fully open your mouth. After a full course of treatment about one in five people find that the range of movement of their jaw is reduced by one-third or more. Doctors call this stiffness and restricted jaw movement trismus. Trismus usually first appears a month or two after the end of a course of radiotherapy, and is likely to get gradually worse for some months, or even years later, but the most noticeable changes have usually happened within nine months of ending treatment.

The pelvis

The bowel

The lower part of the bowel, which runs through the pelvis, is called the rectum, and radiotherapy to the pelvis will make the rectum inflamed. With lower doses this will not really be noticeable but as the dose rises a series of increasingly troublesome problems might develop. To begin with these are likely to be some mild diarrhoea, looseness of the bowels, with discomfort in the back passage (this discomfort can often make it feel as though you want to go to the toilet when actually the bowel is quite empty and you don't need to). As the treatment progresses and the dose rises, about one in three people will go on to get more troublesome problems: the diarrhoea will get worse, becoming more frequent, often with a lot of white slimy mucous being passed as well. Having your bowels open might be quite painful with a gripping, cramping sensation in the back passage (which doctors call tenesmus). Sometimes it is difficult to control the urge to have your bowels open and this can lead to some incontinence with 'accidents'. This more severe diarrhoea is often accompanied by tummy cramps and pains. If the diarrhoea gets really bad then there may be some bleeding from the bowel and blood may appear mixed in with the stools.

These side effects are likely to come on during the second or third week of a high-dose course of treatment to the pelvis and will get progressively worse until two or three weeks after the course has ended, and then gradually settle back to normal over another six to eight weeks. But sometimes there is permanent damage to the rectum which goes on to cause long-term side effects with continuing diarrhoea, passage of mucous, and bleeding from the bowel. For most people who have high-dose radiotherapy to their pelvis these problems, if they do occur, are likely to be mild and not too troublesome, but for about one in twenty people they may be much more severe. There may also be difficulty in controlling bowel movements; this may lead to needing to go to the toilet urgently, with very little warning, or there may be some actual incontinence; there might also be some pain when stools are passed. Sometimes the rectum may become narrowed because of scar tissue forming (fibrosis) and may even become blocked (obstructed), or it might begin to leak internally (perforation of the bowel). These late severe effects are very uncommon but obviously when they do occur they can be very serious and need urgent treatment.

The bladder

The bladder lies low down in the pelvis, just behind the pubic bone and will become inflamed during pelvic radiotherapy; this is called radiation cystitis. Once again troublesome symptoms will only appear with higher doses and will become more severe as the dose increases.

The first symptom is usually the need to pass urine more often than normal (doctors call this frequency). Sometimes there will be some mild stinging or burning in the urethra (the tube which connects the bladder to the outside) as you pass water.

About four out of ten people having higher doses of radiotherapy to their pelvis will go on to get more troublesome problems: the frequency will become more frequent and this often goes along with a sudden uncontrollable urge to pass water, which can often lead to leakage and incontinence of urine. Cramping spasms of pain in the bladder and the pelvis may develop, and at this stage there is often bleeding from the lining of the bladder, so the urine becomes heavily bloodstained, often with the passage of dark clots of blood. These side effects are likely to come on during the second or third week of a high-dose course of treatment to the pelvis and will get progressively worse until two or three weeks after the course has ended, and then gradually settle back to normal over another six to eight weeks. But sometimes there is permanent damage to the bladder leading to long-term problems with frequency, pain and the passage of blood in the urine (haematuria).

Another thing that people often notice when they have radiotherapy to their bladder is that they pass 'bits' in their urine. These are tiny flakes of tissue that look like little grey, pink or white specks in your water. This can be quite worrying but it is perfectly harmless, and not a sign of anything going wrong. This symptom usually disappears on its own within a few weeks of finishing treatment.

Other side effects for men

Radiotherapy to the pelvis may lead to impotence. This is more likely in older men, and with higher doses of treatment. Having other illnesses, such as diabetes, also increases the chances of a loss of potency. Estimates vary, but between one in three and one in five men may find that they are unable to get an erection after a course of radiotherapy to their pelvis.

Irradiation of the prostate gland may also lead to narrowing of the urethra, the tube which passes through the gland, carrying urine from the bladder to the penis. This can lead to difficulty passing urine, with a slow start to peeing, a poor stream and some dribbling of urine afterwards. Occasionally the urethra may actually become blocked because of inflammation and scar tissue, so that it is impossible to pass urine. If this does happen it can usually be sorted out very quickly but it will mean a trip to hospital.

Other side effects for women

The ovaries lie deep in the pelvis and are very sensitive to radiation. This means that most radiotherapy treatments to the pelvis will stop the ovaries working permanently. This means that you will become infertile and will not be able to have children. It also means that as the ovaries are no longer making female hormones, your periods will stop and you will become menopausal. So you will get some or all of the symptoms of the menopause. These may include hot flushes, night sweats, vaginal dryness, mood changes and some irritability, and some difficulty with concentration and loss of memory.

If your pelvic radiotherapy includes your vagina this may lead to a number of problems including soreness and dryness and the risk of narrowing and shortening of the vagina; these can be uncomfortable and may make intercourse quite painful. These symptoms often only become noticeable some weeks or months after you have finished treatment. Soreness and dryness is due to damage to the glands in the lining of your vagina and, depending on the dose of radiation used, these changes may be temporary, lasting a few months, or permanent. Narrowing or shortening of your vagina happens because of the inflammation caused by radiotherapy which leads to scar tissue forming in the walls of your vagina. Also, bands of fibrous tissue may form between the walls of the vagina; these are called adhesions. To begin with these adhesions are very flimsy but with time they thicken and strengthen and can cause discomfort and make intercourse difficult or painful.

Can radiotherapy cause cancer?

We know from studies done following the atomic bomb attacks on Hiroshima and Nagasaki during the Second World War, and from the aftermath of the Chernobyl disaster in the 1980s, that being exposed to ionizing radiation can cause cancer. Does this mean that having radiotherapy, which involves being treated with ionizing radiation, can actually cause cancer as well as curing it?

A lot of research has been done into this subject, and the answer is that having a course of radiotherapy does very slightly increase your chance of getting another cancer. This risk decreases with age, so children or teenagers who have radiotherapy are more likely to get a second cancer as a result of their treatment than adults. Working out the exact risk is difficult, partly because it may take ten or twenty years for a second cancer to develop after radiotherapy, and partly because many people who have never had radiotherapy will go on to get another cancer after they have had a first cancer success-fully treated. It is likely that, for adults, less than 1 in 1000 people who have radiotherapy will get a second cancer as a result of their treatment. Since that radiotherapy was given as part of a life-saving package of therapy for their original cancer, experts are agreed that the benefits of radiation treatment for cancer far outweigh the risks.

10

Coping with side effects

Tiredness and radiation-related fatigue

Tiredness is the commonest side effect of radiotherapy and most people who have a course of treatment lasting more than a week will be affected by it. You may just feel a bit weary and washed out, but sometimes treatment can leave you completely exhausted and drained. Surprisingly, although tiredness is such a common problem there has been very little research into the subject, and many standard textbooks on radiotherapy do not even mention it! In recent years, however, doctors have become more aware that tiredness is a major problem for many people having a long course of radiotherapy, and will now listen sympathetically and do their best to help you cope with it, whereas in the past it was often considered a minor difficulty that you just had to live with.

If you are troubled by loss of energy and weariness, do mention it to your doctors and nurses. If they don't know you have got a problem then they can't do anything to help. Don't be afraid to tell them how you are feeling, don't feel you are being a nuisance or wasting their time. Very often there are quite simple things they can do, and advice they can give, that can make a big difference.

When tiredness is a real problem many people worry that this is a sign of their cancer coming back or getting worse. It is very important to remember that if you are having a course of radio-therapy then the chances are that you will feel quite drained by it. This is very natural; being weary is not a result of anything going wrong either with your treatment or your underlying illness. And remember, too, that although it may last for some time, the tiredness from radiotherapy is temporary and will eventually go away.

What can your doctors and nurses do to help?

First of all your doctors can sort out why you are feeling tired. Of course this may be all due to your treatment, but sometimes there can be other things making you feel low, or making your radiation-related tiredness worse. These are listed here.

- *Anaemia*. It is quite common for people with a cancer to become anaemic, and this makes you feel very tired. A simple blood test, which gives you an answer within five minutes, will tell whether or not this is a problem. If you are anaemic then your doctors will often recommend a blood transfusion. This can be done as an outpatient over a matter of a few hours with little or no risk, and can transform the way you feel almost instantly, restoring energy and vitality. An alternative these days is a course of injections which stimulate your bone marrow to make more red blood cells, correcting the anaemia, although this may take a little longer to work.
- *Infection*. Having a cancer and having radiotherapy can lower your resistance to infection, and if you pick up a bug then this can be very draining. If you have got an infection then usually a short course of antibiotics will put things right.
- *Depression*. Becoming clinically depressed is something that happens to some people as a result either of their cancer or their radiotherapy. Usually this responds very well to routine anti-depressant drugs, and a few weeks of treatment can often make the world of difference.
- *Thyroid function*. Low levels of thyroid hormone are quite common. Very often these do not cause much in the way of problems, but if you are having to cope with the stresses of a cancer and the effects of radiotherapy then this may tip the balance and lead to excessive tiredness. A simple blood test will check on your thyroid activity, and if this is low then tablets of the hormone thyroxine will put the situation right.

Once other things have been excluded, or corrected, your medical team can focus on helping you deal with your tiredness. A lot of this is about understanding what is happening and adjusting your life around it. But before we come to this there are a couple of other things to mention, which your medical team might suggest and which might help. These are given below.

- *Exercise.* It may seem very strange to talk about exercise at a time when you are feeling worn out. But a number of research studies have shown that taking some regular exercise can help reduce the feeling of tiredness associated with cancer and its treatment. This doesn't mean working out in the gym or running the half-marathon, but if you can manage a gentle walk of about half an hour each day, or a similar level of some other activity, like swimming or cycling, then this will often make quite a difference to the way you feel.
- *Cognitive behaviour therapy.* This involves sessions with a trained therapist or counsellor who works with you to look at your feelings and beliefs about your tiredness. By exploring, and sometimes challenging, those emotions, the therapy can help to alter your mental approach. Once again, research trials have shown that this can be helpful, but unfortunately cognitive behaviour therapy is not widely available on the NHS in the UK.
- *Drugs.* Occasionally your specialist may feel that a course of tablets for a week or two might help. The most widely used drugs are hormones, using either steroids (usually prednisolone or dexamethasone), or progestogens (usually Megace or Provera). These will often improve your appetite, increase your energy levels and give you a general feeling of well-being. These benefits can often be gained with relatively low doses of the drugs, which, during the few weeks they are usually prescribed, should not cause any undue side effects.
- *Support.* Your nurses and doctors can often organize help for you with a number of things, for example arranging transport from home to hospital for your treatment, working with social services to send someone in to do cleaning and housework, working with your GP and the local hospice to give you more nursing and emotional support from home-care teams and community nurses, and arranging financial help and sorting out benefits.

How can you help yourself?

The first thing is to try not to worry. Remember, feeling tired during a course of radiotherapy is extremely common and very natural. Most people having radiotherapy for more than a week or two will feel weary. So being run down, feeling worn out, is not a sign of anything going wrong and does not mean that your treatment is not working – it is simply your body's way of adjusting to what is happening. And things will get better once your treatment is over. The change won't be immediate, but in the weeks after radiotherapy you will gradually notice that life is getting back to a more normal pattern. So your tiredness, your exhaustion, is only temporary; things will improve, you will be your old self again; it is a matter of trying to adjust your life for a few weeks or months, during and after your radiation treatment.

These are a few of the things you might like to think about for trying to cope with the effects of your radiotherapy.

- Don't try and force yourself to carry on as normal. Look at what you do during the day; work out those things that have to be done and those that you can put to one side. Focus on the essentials and keep everything else to a minimum.
- If you feel like having a rest, stopping and putting your feet up, then do. Struggling to do things when you feel exhausted won't help, whereas sitting down for half an hour, or having a short nap, might make all the difference.
- Don't give up completely. Try and find one or two light chores or easy tasks that you can manage to keep you in touch with your normal routine, without overdoing things.
- Try and find time for a bit of gentle exercise.
- See if you can find things that will distract you from thinking about your tiredness, your treatment and your cancer: favourite TV programmes, the radio, a good book, crossword puzzles or Sudoku, the letters you were always going to write but never had time for, the phone calls to friends and relatives you can never normally fit in.
- Don't be afraid to accept offers of help from family, friends and neighbours: offers of a lift to hospital for your treatment, or looking after the children for an afternoon, or coming in and

cooking lunch – every little helps, and they will usually get a lot of pleasure and satisfaction from feeling they are helping you.

- Don't be afraid to ask for help if you need it. People will usually be very sympathetic and supportive, and you are only going to need their help for a while until things get better.
- If you are struggling then do let your doctors or nurses know; there is a lot they can do to help but they can only do this if they know you need them.

Skin changes

Following a few simple guidelines can help reduce your chances of getting sore and inflamed skin in the area that is being treated. For many years the routine advice was that you should never wash the skin that was being irradiated, but with modern-day treatment this is no longer the case and it is quite OK to wash, shower or bath. However, there is still quite a long list of dos and don'ts to try and remember:

- wash the treated skin every day;
- use warm or tepid water with an unperfumed soap (chemists and most supermarkets will stock natural soaps without additives);
- if you are showering, avoid very powerful jets of water;
- don't use perfumed products, aftershave or deodorant on the treated skin;
- when you are washing avoid rubbing the area with a flannel or washcloth;
- use a soft towel to pat the skin dry, rather than rubbing it – the friction will irritate your skin;
- if you want to use any gels or creams on your skin check with your treatment team to make sure they are safe;
- if you are a man and treatment includes the skin of your face then use an electric razor for shaving rather than a wet shave;
- if treatment includes your armpit (axilla) then avoid shaving this area;
- don't use hair-removing creams or waxing to remove hair in the treatment area;

- wear lose clothing made of natural fibres to keep friction to the treated skin to a minimum;
- use a mild detergent to wash clothes that will be in contact with the treated skin;
- try not to scratch or rub your skin;
- avoid using any sticky tapes or plasters on the treated skin until any reaction to your treatment has completely settled;
- sunlight will probably make skin soreness more likely, so if you are out in the sun keep the treated area covered until your course of treatment has finished and any skin reaction has completely settled.

Once your treatment is over and any soreness and inflammation has settled completely, then you can generally go back to your normal routine. But for at least a year after treatment the skin that has been irradiated will be more sensitive than normal to sunlight, so if you are out in the sun, and your treated skin is going to be exposed, then use a sunblock of at least SPF 15 to protect against sunburn.

Radiotherapy does tend to dry your skin, and many treatment centres recommend routinely using a moisturizing cream during your course of treatment. Check with your treatment team to see whether they think this would be a good idea for you, and get their advice as to the best cream to use. Incidentally, people sometimes ask if it is all right to go swimming while you are having radiotherapy. Generally the answer is yes, but one thing to remember is that the chlorine in swimming pools tends to dry your skin, so once again using a moisturizer might be a good idea.

These fairly straightforward precautions should help reduce your risk of getting skin soreness during radiotherapy, but with some treatments some degree of skin reaction is still virtually unavoidable. The radiotherapists (therapy radiographers) who supervise your treatment each time you come will keep a watch for any signs of your skin becoming inflamed, but if you are getting problems do let them know and get their advice.

In general terms, when skin changes are mild with just some reddening (erythema) and slight irritation or soreness, using a soothing cream like E45 or Unguentum Merck is often helpful. If the irritation is more troublesome, and these are not helping then a mild steroid cream, such as hydrocortisone 1 per cent can often give a lot of relief.

If the changes become worse and the skin blisters and peels, leaving a red moist surface in places (moist desquamation) then creams should not be used, but sometimes special dressings such as hydrogels and siliconized gel dressings can speed up the healing and make things more comfortable.

When the skin is raw and moist it makes a clear fluid discharge. If this discharge changes colour and becomes yellow or green, often becoming very smelly as well, then this is a sign that the area has become infected and a special dressing impregnated with antibacterial agents may be needed, sometimes together with a course of antibiotic tablets or capsules, in order to clear up the infection.

Usually, even with quite severe skin reactions all the changes will settle down within a few weeks of finishing your radiotherapy and things will get more or less back to normal. But sometimes, especially with higher doses, the skin in the treated area may be permanently a bit drier and thinner than the surrounding areas, and using a moisturizing cream long term may be necessary to keep things comfortable. Also any skin that has received a course of radiotherapy will always be more sensitive to sunlight, and so if you are going to be out in the sunshine and the part of your body that has been treated is going to be exposed then do use a sun block of at least SPF 15 strength to protect it.

Mouth problems

Radiotherapy can affect your mouth in several ways. Sometimes it can cause soreness of the inside of your mouth. If this happens, it usually comes on a week or so after you have started your treatment. When you look in your mouth there may be nothing to see, or there may be some redness of the lining of your mouth (the mucosa), and sometimes there may be small ulcers. This inflammation and soreness of the lining of the mouth is called mucositis.

Sometimes you may also get an infection in your mouth. The most common type of infection is called thrush (also known as oral candidiasis, or oral monilia). This usually shows up as small whitish patches on the mucosa and the surface of the tongue. Another quite common problem with radiotherapy is getting a dry mouth, because the treatment stops your salivary glands from working properly. This can also lead to changes of taste, with some foods and drinks tasting different from normal.

Usually the mucositis associated with radiotherapy will last for up to two or three weeks after your treatment is over; once it starts to improve the recovery is usually very quick, over a matter of just a few days. Depending on the dose of radiation you have had your salivary glands will often recover and start working again about three to four months after your treatment has ended, but sometimes, with high-dose treatments, a dry mouth may be a longer-term or even a permanent problem.

A sore mouth

The chances of getting a sore mouth do vary depending on your treatment; some drugs, or combinations of drugs, are more likely to cause mucositis than others. Usually your doctors or nurses will warn you if oral soreness is likely to happen, but if they don't mention it, then you can always ask them about it. If it has been flagged up as a possible side effect, there are a number of things you can do that will help reduce the chances of it developing.

- Have a routine check-up with your dentist before you start treatment, just to be sure there are no obvious tooth or gum problems that need to be dealt with before your radiotherapy.
- Rinse your mouth three or four times a day with a salt solution: use two teaspoonfuls of salt to a pint of water, then boil this mixture to dissolve the salt and sterilize the water, let it cool and store it in your fridge.
- Keep up good oral hygiene; this means cleaning your teeth at least twice a day. Using a normal toothbrush can be uncomfortable, so using a soft toothbrush or a child's brush might help. You may find that your usual toothpaste makes your mouth and gums sore, and changing to a brand for 'sensitive teeth', like Sensodyne Original or Macleans Sensitive, might help. Mouthwashes can also be useful, and you can try these

if you find that brushing your teeth is really painful. There are preparations you can get from your chemist or supermarket that help to prevent infection; these include chlorhexidine, Corsodyl, and thymol. Keeping your mouth moist is a good idea and some tips on how to do this are given later in the section called 'A dry mouth'.

- Change your diet. There are some foods and drinks that can make your mouth sore if the mucosa is sensitive. These include very hot and spicy foods, toast, crisps, vinegar, salt, neat spirits (whisky, brandy, gin, etc.) and acid drinks like grapefruit juice and some types of orange juice – so avoiding these might be a good idea.

If you get a sore mouth, then do mention it to your radiographers or doctors. They will be able to check for signs of infection and give you advice on what to do. If you have got thrush, then this is easily treated by a course of an antifungal drug like nystatin or amphotericin for a few days. These drugs are given either as a pastille to suck four times a day or as a mouthwash that you rinse round your mouth and then swallow four times a day. If there is no evidence of infection, then these are some of the other things you can do to help a sore mouth during your radiotherapy.

- Use a painkilling mouthwash. Difflam Oral Rinse is a mouthwash you can buy over the counter which can help. It is also available as a spray. Some people find using the full-strength mouthwash stings, and diluting it with an equal amount of warm water may help. An alternative is to make your own mouthwash using soluble aspirin, dissolving a couple of tablets in a glass of warm water and using this to rinse your mouth well three or four times a day.
- If you have mouth ulcers, then there is a wide range of gels, pastes and sprays that you can get that might help. These include Bonjela gel, Biora gel, Medijel, Rinstead contact pastilles, and many more. Your local pharmacist will always be able to advise you on what is available.
- Sometimes taking a mild painkiller can be helpful. Paracetamol capsules or soluble paracetamol tablets, taken two or three times daily, may reduce your discomfort.

A dry mouth

If you get a dry mouth during or after your treatment, there are a number of things that might help.

- Keep your mouth moist with regular fluids. You should be drinking at least two litres (four pints) of fluid every day during your treatment, but supplementing this with regular sips of water or other soft drinks can help (fizzy water, or other fizzy drinks, tend to be better than still fluids). Sucking ice cubes or crushed ice is another idea.
- Smearing the surface of your tongue and the lining of your mouth with a little olive oil or melted butter will keep things moist for a while and is often particularly effective last thing at night.
- Chewing sugar-free chewing gum, or sugar-free fruit pastilles, can help stimulate your salivary glands to make moisture for your mouth. In the same way, sucking pineapple chunks may help.
- Cleaning your mouth regularly with baking soda (sodium bicarbonate) mouthwashes (one teaspoonful of powder in a glass of warm water) keeps the mucosa moist and clean.
- Drinking a glass of sherry (especially dry, rather than medium or sweet sherry) about a quarter of an hour before a meal can often stimulate the salivary glands, and your digestive system, to make eating easier and more appealing.
- Moistening your food helps, using plenty of gravy or sauces. On the other hand, dry foods are best avoided, especially things like crackers, flaky pastry and chocolate, which all tend to stick to the lining of your mouth.
- There are a number of over-the-counter preparations of artificial saliva that some people find useful. These may come as sprays, gels, pastilles or tablets, and include Saliva Orthana, Glandosane, Luborant, Saliveze, Salivix and SST. Once again, your local pharmacist will be happy to advise you on what is available.
- Using a lip balm to moisten your lips and keep them soft might make a difference.
- There are also some things to try to avoid. Smoking, alcohol and caffeine (in tea and coffee) all tend to make your mouth dry, so cutting back on these is a good thing.

Jaw stiffness

If your radiotherapy treatment covered the hinge joint just in front of your ears (the temporomandibular joint), which controls the opening and shutting of your mouth, then this may stiffen the muscles and tissues around the joint, leading to stiffness and difficulty in fully opening your mouth. This stiffness of the jaw is called trismus.

People having radiotherapy that covers their jaw joint will usually be given advice about regular exercises, and possibly massage as well, to help prevent the problem of trismus developing. If jaw stiffness does develop then there are a number of ways to try and help, which are based on stretching the jaw. These range from the relatively simple method of sliding wooden spatulas, or tongue depressors, between the upper and lower front teeth to move the jaws apart, gradually increasing the number of spatulas over a period of time so that the angle of mouth widening is steadily increased, to a more sophisticated and possibly more successful version of this approach – a simple machine called the Therabite, which can be used regularly and simply, fitting over the upper and lower teeth and then gently stretching the jaw.

Difficulty swallowing food

If you are having radiotherapy to the centre of your chest or to your neck, the inflammation that develops in your gullet (oesophagus) during treatment may make it difficult for you to swallow food (doctors call this dysphagia). There are a number of things you can try to help ease this problem:

- eat little and often rather than two or three big meals each day;
- make sure you are sitting up straight when you are eating;
- try and be as relaxed and quiet as possible when you are eating;
- yawning a few times before you start to eat can help relax your throat muscles;
- take small mouthfuls and chew your food very well before you swallow;
- keep your food moist, either by taking sips of water while you are eating, or by using plenty of gravy, sauces, custard and cream;

- liquidize your food in a blender in order to make thick soups or smoothies;
- cold foods, like ice cream and yoghurts, are often easier to manage and more soothing than hot foods;
- avoid dry or rough foods, like toast, pastry, crisps.

If swallowing food is painful then your oncologists should be able to prescribe painkilling medicines which will help make things more comfortable. They will often also be able to arrange for you to see a dietitian to get their advice on coping with your dysphagia.

Very occasionally, swallowing can get so difficult that it is hard even to manage liquids. This is obviously very frightening and upsetting. It is usually only a short-term problem while the inflammation from the radiotherapy is at its worst. To tide you through this period your specialist may recommend something called PEG feeding. The initials stand for percutaneous endoscopic gastrostomy. This involves having a small operation to put a tube through the front of your belly into your stomach so that specially prepared liquids containing all the nutrients you need can be put through this, bypassing your gullet. Although this sounds rather alarming the operation is very quick, simple and safe, and does not even need a general anaesthetic. When the tube is in place and you have got used to it then you can be up and about and carry on with life. Once your swallowing begins to get better the tube can be removed and you can get back to normal eating and drinking.

Diet supplements

If you are having difficulty eating or swallowing as result of your radiotherapy, or if you are just feeling off your food and unable to face your normal meals, then nutritional supplements may help to give you all the dietary essentials that you are missing. There are a wide range of products that you can get as nutritional supplements. Many of these are things that you can buy over the counter at chemists or supermarkets, although some can be expensive. There are fortified soups and puddings, as well as powders like Complan or Build-up, which come in a range of flavours and are mixed with milk to make a nutritious drink.

There are also a range of supplements that you can get on prescription, which may be much cheaper. These include a number of liquids which come in tetrapak cartons, bottles or bags, such as Ensure plus (which has a mix of protein, fat and carbohydrate), Enrich plus (which has a similar mix of nutrients with additional fibre), Enlive plus (which is fat-free) and Fortisip and Fresubin which come in several versions, each with a different mix of nutrients. Ensure plus also comes in the form of a yoghurt. All these come in a range of flavours. There is also Maxijul, which is mainly carbohydrate and comes in both liquid and powder forms.

Most radiotherapy departments will have a dietitian as part of the team, and if you feel your diet needs a boost do mention it to your oncologist or radiographers and they should be able to arrange an appointment for you to get expert advice on which supplements would be best for you.

Breathlessness and cough

If your course of radiotherapy involved treatment to some of your chest then you may notice some shortness of breath and/or a dry cough coming on a few weeks after your treatment has finished. This might be due to parts of your lungs being inflamed by the radiation (doctors call this radiation pneumonitis). However, there are many other reasons why breathlessness or a cough might occur, so if you are feeling short-winded after your treatment the first thing to do is to let your doctors know, and they can then find out the cause of the problem. Usually a simple chest X-ray is all that is needed to make the diagnosis of radiation pneumonitis.

If your symptoms are due to radiotherapy they will usually disappear on their own over a matter of a few weeks. If you have mild breathlessness, which you only notice when you are very active, or if your cough is slight and occasional, then the reassurance of knowing what is wrong, and the knowledge that it will get better soon, is often the only 'treatment' that is needed. But if your symptoms are more troublesome then a course of steroid tablets, like prednisolone, for a few weeks should give more or less complete relief. Usually the doses of steroid that are needed are fairly small, so there shouldn't be any unpleasant side effects.

Sickness: nausea and vomiting

If sickness does develop while you are having radiotherapy it is usually not very severe, nothing like as bad as the nausea and vomiting that can happen with some types of chemotherapy. This means that often quite a mild anti-sickness tablet will be enough to control the problem for you and make life comfortable again. Commonly used medications are Maxolon (metoclopramide), Motilium (domperidone) and Stemetil (prochlorperazine). Very occasionally these will not be sufficient to ease the symptoms and you may need a stronger drug like Zofran (ondansetron) or Kytril (granisetron). It would be very unusual for one of these drugs not to help, but if you are still having problems then combining them with a steroid tablet, like dexamethasone, should help. Even if you don't feel like eating because of feeling sick it is still important to try and keep drinking and take in at least two litres of fluid each day.

Diarrhoea

If you are having radiotherapy to your pelvis then it is likely that the treatment will include all or part of the lower part of your large bowel, the rectum, and this may well lead to some diarrhoea. This is likely to come on gradually a week or so after you have started treatment. Often making a few simple changes to your diet at the first sign of any looseness of your bowels can nip the problem in the bud. If you find you are needing to have your bowels open more often, or your motions are becoming more liquid, then a change in diet can help. The advice is to eat what these days we would think of as a rather unhealthy choice of foods, cutting out fruit and green vegetables, avoiding brown bread and any other high-fibre items. Your radiographers should be able to give you a diet sheet with advice about what you should and shouldn't be eating. Taking plenty of fluids is important, so that you don't get dehydrated; aim for at least two litres a day, and ideally more. Water is probably the best drink but other things are OK, apart from fruit juice, which can tend to make diarrhoea worse. If a change in diet doesn't help then your doctor can always give you tablets or capsules that can ease the problem. Either Imodium (loperamide) or Lomotil (co-phenotrope) are usually the first line of treatment, but if the diarrhoea gets very troublesome, which is unusual, then you may need a stronger drug: codeine phosphate.

Bladder problems

Radiotherapy to the bladder can cause troublesome symptoms like passing urine more often (frequency), needing to pass water very urgently (urgency), and stinging or burning when you pee (dysuria). Drinking plenty of water can help reduce the risk of getting these symptoms and help ease them if they do develop – this might seem strange when passing water very often is part of the problem, but keeping your bladder flushed through helps to remove impurities which can make the irritation worse. Also, drinking a glass of cranberry juice once a day can help prevent infections of your bladder and may soothe the inflammation from the radiation.

Infection of the bladder is quite common during radiotherapy, and the symptoms of radiation side effects are very like those of an infection. If you get problems with your waterworks while you are having treatment do let your radiographers or doctors know. They can then arrange a simple urine test to check for infection. If there is a bug then a course of antibiotics will usually put things right in a few days.

For mild bladder discomfort your doctors may suggest taking potassium citrate mixture (sometimes called mist. pot. cit.). This lowers the level of acid in your urine, and thus reduces the irritation to the lining of your bladder. For more severe discomfort your clinical oncologist may suggest taking anti-inflammatory tablets, or might prescribe drugs which help to relax the muscles in your bladder and ease painful bladder spasms.

Incidentally, there is some evidence that acupuncture can help ease bladder discomfort during radiotherapy, but unfortunately this is not widely available on the NHS.

Additional problems for men

Sometimes after a course of radiotherapy to your pelvis you may find it difficult to get an erection; this may or may not go together with a loss of interest in sex generally. This may have a variety of causes, which may be both emotional and physical. Anxiety and depression can both play a part here, and once again just talking about and understanding the problem may make a difference, and adjusting your love-making to a pattern where you need more time, encouragement and stimulation than before might make a difference. If depression is a problem, then antidepressants may help. If there is a more physical basis for the difficulty, as a result of either the treatment given or the effects of the cancer itself, then drugs like sildenafil (Viagra), vardenafil (Levitra) or tadalafil (Cialis) may help. These are only available on prescription so you would need to discuss this with your doctor. Other solutions for physical problems include small injections of drugs like papavarine or alprostadil (Caverjet, Viridal), which you can be taught to give as injections directly into the penis, or, in the case of alprostadil, alternatively as pellets inserted into the penis.

Another approach is the use of vacuum pumps, which can be applied to the penis before intercourse to stimulate an erection. Sorting out the right approach to this problem can be difficult and it is something where you probably need to talk to your doctor to get his or her advice on what can be done to help.

As already mentioned, depression can be a cause of loss of interest in sex at this time. Feeling low and miserable at times while you are having radiotherapy is very understandable, but for some people this tips over into clinical depression, which becomes a more constant problem where your mood is low all the time and nothing and nobody seems to be able to cheer you up; life just seems pointless and hopeless. A loss of sex drive is almost always part of the picture of clinical depression. If this describes the way you are feeling, then discuss things with your family doctor or hospital specialist because there are very good drugs that can be given to treat clinical depression, and the benefits can often be rapid and dramatic. This is not a problem that you should suffer, when such easy, safe and effective help is available.

Another problem may be difficulty in passing urine; you may find that you are slow to start, or have only a very weak stream and take a long time, often with some dribbling of urine afterwards. This is often due to narrowing of the urethra because of scarring from the radiotherapy. Usually the problem can be solved quite easily by a urethral dilation. This is done at hospital, either as a day-patient or with an overnight stay. You will be given an anaesthetic and then special probes will be passed into your urethra to stretch it and open up the narrowed channel. Although this sounds painful, as you are asleep you won't feel anything and it can make an immediate difference.

If the narrowing of the urethra becomes so severe that it is actually blocked, and you cannot pass water at all (doctors call this urinary retention), then you will need to go to hospital and the doctors will pass a soft, flexible tube (catheter) through your urethra, into your bladder, to allow the urine to drain away. This can be done without an anaesthetic and gives huge relief in a matter of moments. This may solve the problem, and the catheter can be removed shortly afterwards, or you may need to go on to have a urethral dilation. Very occasionally it will be necessary to keep the catheter in on a long-term basis. If this happens the catheter is attached to a drainage bag, which is usually strapped to your thigh and which you can empty as and when necessary.

Additional problems for women

Managing menopausal symptoms

For many younger women who have pelvic radiotherapy coping with menopausal symptoms can be a big problem. The main problem is hot flushes, which often occur along with drenching sweats, palpitations and feelings of anxiety or irritability, all of which can be very upsetting. These symptoms all relate to suppression of the ovaries and there are a number of ways to try and help.

Sometimes simple lifestyle changes make things easier. Taking regular exercise, losing some weight and avoiding getting too hot might help. Also some women find that certain foods, particularly spicy foods, and certain drinks, particularly alcohol, act as triggers to bring on their flushes, and avoiding these can also reduce the problem.

Many women turn to complementary therapies. There are a number of preparations available from pharmacists and health food shops which contain plant oestrogens (phyto-oestrogens) which may help. The active ingredients include red clover, soy, genistein and black cohosh. Vitamin E supplements have also been shown to help in some studies. Although they are quite popular, and many women feel they make a difference, scientific studies suggest that neither evening primrose oil nor ginseng reduce the number and severity of hot flushes and sweats.

Another approach is to try either acupuncture or relaxation therapies. Studies have shown that both of these techniques can help some women.

Sometimes prescription drugs may improve the situation. The options here include low doses of the female hormone progesterone, certain types of antidepressants, and a drug called clonidine that alters the blood vessels to reduce flushes and sweats. None of these is an absolutely sure way of improving the problem, but if the symptoms are severe and troublesome they might be worth a try, and it would be a good idea to have a word with your doctors and see what they think.

As the whole problem is the result of treatment bringing on the menopause it might seem logical to try HRT (hormone replacement therapy). This is often very effective at relieving the symptoms, but there have been worries that it might increase the risk of getting breast cancer. However, this only seems to be likely in older women who take HRT after their natural menopause; so certainly for women up to the age of 50 it is quite all right to take HRT. An alternative to standard hormone replacement therapy might be the drug tibilone, which has some oestrogen-like activity and seems as effective as HRT in easing flushes and sweats.

If vaginal dryness is a problem then there are a number of solutions. There are a variety of lubricants which you can buy at chemists or supermarkets which you and your partner can use. These include KY jelly, Senselle, Sylk and Astroglide, or simple glycerine can be used as an alternative, although unlike the others it is not water soluble and so is a bit more sticky. Another alternative is Replens, which again can be bought over the counter. This is a gel which is a longer-acting vaginal moisturizer, and if used three times a week can help to overcome vaginal dryness and irritation. There are also creams or gels for vaginal use which you can only get on prescription. These contain small amounts of the female hormone oestrogen which nourishes the lining of the vagina and makes it more moist. These include Vagifem, Ovestin, Premarin and Ortho-Gynest. So if vaginal discomfort is a problem do talk to your medical team about it.

Vaginal narrowing or shortening

A build-up of scar tissue in its walls can cause narrowing and shortening of your vagina in the weeks and months after treatment, and this problem is often increased by the formation of adhesions, bands of scar tissue between the walls of the vagina. Regular use of a dilator can usually prevent these problems developing and becoming troublesome. All women who are having radiotherapy that includes their vagina should be given advice about using a dilator. These are usually made of plastic and shaped like a tampon. They come in a variety of widths and lengths. It is best to start using them about two weeks after completing your radiotherapy. The dilators come with a special lubricant which makes it easy to slide them in and the usual advice is to try and hold them inside you for between five and fifteen minutes. To begin with they should be inserted twice a day, for about six weeks, then three times a week for the next six months, and about once a week after that. Having regular sexual intercourse acts a bit like using a dilator, helping to stretch your vagina and break down any adhesions and scar tissue. But even if you are having regular sex, using a dilator is still a good idea to make sure that you don't develop problems from scar tissue forming. Your radiographers or nurses should give you clear and detailed advice about using dilators.

11

Radiotherapy and everyday life

Almost everyone who has radiotherapy will do so as part of their treatment for a cancer. The actual impact of radiotherapy on everyday life is very variable – some people might only have a single treatment, which will hardly affect them at all, while others might have a course of therapy over six to eight weeks, with considerable side effects that may alter their everyday lives for weeks or months afterwards. Furthermore, many people will have radiotherapy as part of a package of treatment, along with either chemotherapy or surgery or both of these. As a consequence of all this it is very often impossible to separate out how much of the way your life changes is just because of the radiotherapy and how much of the way you think and feel is due to knowing you have had cancer, and the disturbance caused by other treatments you have had to go through. So this chapter is about how to handle the impact of the whole cancer experience on the way you live, rather than trying just to single out the effects of your radiation treatment, although where there are specific things to say about this they will be mentioned.

Getting to hospital

Some people say that the most stressful part of their radiotherapy was finding somewhere to park each day when they came for their treatment. Unfortunately this can often be a problem. To make matters worse in most hospitals where there are parking spots near to the radiotherapy department you will have to pay to use them. Allow plenty of time for getting to hospital, and parking, each day; but if you are late, your radiographers will understand and will still give you your treatment. When it comes to paying for parking, the rules and the charges vary from hospital to hospital. Most will allow you free parking if you have a blue 'disabled' sticker, although the number of parking places may be limited. Many hospitals also offer weekly or monthly season tickets that greatly reduce the cost of parking if you are coming for regular visits for a course of radiotherapy. Check with your radiographers what the local arrangements are, and whether there are any special deals that can reduce the charges for you.

If you don't have a car, and have a difficult journey by public transport, or if you don't feel well enough to drive yourself and can't find anybody to bring you for your treatment, most radiotherapy centres can arrange hospital transport to get you there. This may involve a hospital car or a sitting ambulance (which can usually accommodate wheelchairs if necessary). This service is free on the NHS, but it can involve quite a lot of waiting around to be picked up and taken home, and you may go by quite a roundabout route to collect or drop off other people on the way.

Work and radiotherapy

One of the commonest of all radiotherapy treatments is irradiation of the breast after surgery for breast cancer. In the UK this usually involves a three- to four-week course of treatment (although in other countries it may be longer), and moderate doses of radiation are used. Some research has been done to look at the effect of this kind of treatment on women's working lives. These are some of the results from that study:

- about 1 in 5 women were able to carry on working normally throughout their treatment and in the months afterwards;
- about 2 out of 3 women were back at work within six months of finishing radiotherapy;
- about 4 out of 5 women were back at work within one year of finishing radiotherapy;
- these numbers were very similar for women working part-time and full-time;
- about 1 in 3 women reduced their hours of work after their treatment;
- older women were less likely than younger women to carry on working normally.

For people having shorter courses and lower doses of radiotherapy their working lives are likely to be less affected, but with higher doses and longer courses the impact may well be greater and more long-lasting. So for some people radiotherapy will mean little or no change to their jobs, while for others it will make a huge difference. So if you are working and facing the prospect of having radiotherapy, then you need to think ahead about how this will affect your job. In order to help your planning you will need to know some basic facts about your cancer and its treatment. So you should ask your doctors and nurses some of the following questions.

- How long will the radiotherapy go on for?
- What will be involved, in terms of the number and frequency of hospital visits?
- What are the likely side effects, how troublesome might they be, and how long are they going to last?
- What is the likely outcome of the treatment: will the cancer probably be cured completely, or is the radiotherapy being given to try and control it for a period of time before it comes back again?

And, of course, you can get their advice on how easy, or difficult, they feel it might be for you to carry on working during treatment.

Once you have got this information you can start to think about what you personally would like to do with respect to your job. For some people, work is the most important thing in their lives and they would do anything possible to avoid having time off. For others, work is a drudge and a chore, and the chance to give it up, even for a while, would be a real bonus. Also, for some people, the diagnosis of cancer, and its treatment, might give them the opportunity for early retirement, or retirement on the grounds of ill health, and this may be something else you might want to think about.

When you have got an idea of how you would like to handle your working life during, and immediately after, radiotherapy, the next thing is to talk to your employer about the options available. Most employers will be sympathetic in this situation and try and make arrangements for things like time off, flexible working hours, lighter duties, or working from home. If your workplace has an occupational health department or a human resources team then chatting to them can often give you a good idea of the choices open to you. They will be able to tell you about your company's sickness policies and your entitlements to sick leave and pay during that time. They will also treat their discussions with you in strict confidence.

Most employers are very supportive of staff who develop cancer and need radiotherapy. But if you do have problems, then you do also have rights. Most people with cancer will be covered by the Disability Discrimination Act. This Act says that it is unlawful for an employer to discriminate against a person because of their disability. To be classed as 'disabled' under the Act, someone with cancer must have symptoms, or side effects of treatment, that interfere with their day-to-day activities. So if the effects of your radiotherapy mean that your treatment will limit or prevent your ability to work, then you should be covered. The Act also covers people who have recovered from a disability, so if you have been cured as a result of your treatment, your employer cannot discriminate against you because you have had cancer in the past.

Under the terms of the Act, an employer should make 'reasonable adjustments' to workplaces and working practices to make sure that you are not at any substantial disadvantage compared to your colleagues at work. The phrase 'reasonable adjustments' would usually cover things like time off for hospital visits, changes in your working hours, avoiding physically demanding jobs, or allowing a gradual return to work after a period of sick leave.

If you feel your supervisors or managers are being unreasonable or unhelpful, then you could talk to your occupational health or human resources team at work. If you need advice outside of your workplace, then you could talk to your union representative or contact your local Citizens Advice Bureau. Very occasionally, it may even help to get guidance from a lawyer.

Financial help

Sometimes being on radiotherapy, and the time you need to recover afterwards, can lead to some financial hardship, and there are a number of state benefits that are on offer to help during this period.

They are there for the asking, so do not hesitate to apply if you feel they would help you.

The main benefits are listed here.

- *Disability Living Allowance (DLA).* This allowance is for anyone under 65 who needs help with their day-to-day care because of their illness. A special category within this allowance is called 'special rules', and this is for anyone who is unlikely to live longer than six months. A 'special rules' payment means you get the highest rate of payment possible, your claim is given priority and payment is made immediately. Although the 'special rules' do say they are for people with a life expectancy of six months or less, most people who have an advanced (incurable) cancer will find that they are able to get this allowance, even if they live considerably longer than six months. Anyone is entitled to this allowance, regardless of their income or savings, and it is tax-free.
- *Attendance Allowance (AA).* This allowance is similar to the Disability Living Allowance, but is for people of 65 or over. Like the Disability Living Allowance, the Attendance Allowance is not means-tested and is not taxable.
- *Invalid Carer's Allowance (ICA).* This is a payment to carers. To qualify you have to be over 16, you must not earn more than £79 a week, and you cannot claim any other benefits. Also, the person you care for must be receiving Attendance Allowance or Disability Living Allowance Care Component.

Other government benefits that may help include: Income Support (if you are aged between 18 and 60 and are working less than 16 hours a week); Working Tax Credit (if you are on a low income); Pension Credit (if you are over 60 and on a low income); and Child Tax Credit (if you have dependent children). Also, if you are already claiming Income Support you may be able to get help with your mortgage repayments if you need this.

Another type of support is the Direct Payment scheme. This gives cash to people who need to employ someone to help with their care. This can include making payments to a close relative, provided that they do not live with you. This scheme is run by your local council-run social services and is separate from the government benefits, which are paid by the Department of Works and Pensions. So even if you have one of the DWP benefits, you can still contact your local social services department to ask about Direct Payments.

In addition to these various state allowances, the charity Macmillan Cancer Relief does give financial grants to cancer patients who are in need. You can apply for these to cover various living expenses or for things like a special holiday.

Holidays and travel

It is unlikely that you will want to have a holiday while you are actually having your course of radiotherapy but people often want to have a break once their treatment is over. If you are planning in advance then it is usually best to allow four to six weeks after the end of your treatment to give time for any immediate side effects to settle down (your doctors should be able to give you an idea of how likely side effects are with your particular treatment, and how troublesome they may be and how long they are likely to last). Once any side effects have eased then your radiation treatment should not restrict your travel plans. However, there could be problems if you are continuing treatment with chemotherapy, or if your cancer is still present and active. If this is the case, and you are thinking of taking a short break somewhere in Britain, this is usually fairly straightforward, but a holiday abroad may be more difficult.

For a trip within the UK, the first thing to do is to check with your doctors and nurses that they think it will be safe for you to do this and that it won't interfere with any treatment or tests that you need. Once you have their agreement, then the two things you need to make sure of are that you take a good supply of all the medicines you need, or might need, with you and that you have some written information about your cancer and its treatment. This is a wise precaution because if you were to be taken ill, and had difficulty in getting straight back to your own hospital, then the doctors where you were staying would need to have details about your condition and the drugs you were having so they could take care of you.

Holidays abroad present more problems. Even if your medical team are happy for you to travel overseas you may have difficulty in getting travel insurance. Most insurers will be reluctant to issue cover to people who are having chemotherapy, or who are within a month or so of having completed their treatment. Some insurers also refuse cover if you have recently had a blood transfusion. It is worth shopping around, however, because companies do vary and you may find that you can get cover, although you may have to pay a premium, and they might also want a report from your doctor confirming that it is all right for you to go abroad. Getting insurance is often easier if you are travelling to countries within the EU, or certain other countries that have reciprocal health agreements with the UK, which means that any treatment you have there would either be free or relatively cheap. By contrast, countries where health costs are much higher, like the USA, can be more difficult to get insurance for.

If you are going abroad, even if you have got insurance, there are a few other things to bear in mind.

- As with trips within the UK, taking written details of your cancer and its treatment is essential.
- Take a good supply of any drugs you need (and take some extra in case of delays on your journey). If you have drugs that have to be given by injection, using needles and syringes, or if you are taking narcotic drugs like morphine, then you may need special permission from the immigration services of the place you are going to, and special documents from your own doctors. Your travel company should be able to advise you, or you could contact the embassy of the country you are hoping to visit.
- Many people with cancer have a higher than normal risk of deep vein thrombosis, and this risk is further increased if you are on certain drugs, like tamoxifen. So if you are going on a long-haul flight, check with your doctors to see whether they feel you are at risk, and what precautions you ought to take.
- If you are hoping to go somewhere where you need vaccinations, this could be a problem. Many people with cancer have reduced immunity, either because of their underlying cancer or the treatment they have had. This means that some vaccines

might actually be dangerous and others could be ineffective. Once again, have a chat with your doctor if you are going to need vaccinations.

Sex

Sex is a sensitive and very personal subject. This means it is often something that people who are going to have radiotherapy feel shy about discussing with their doctors and nurses. Because it is not talked about very much, people do often worry, so it is important to start by stating a few facts.

First, no one can catch cancer from someone else by having sex with them. So there is no risk that you could pass on your cancer to your partner by carrying on with your normal love life.

Second, having sex does not make the cancer worse, or, if it has already been treated successfully, increase the risk of it coming back.

Third, having sex won't interfere with your radiotherapy. It won't stop it from working or make it any less effective or increase the risk of side effects.

Finally, people worry that the treatment makes them radioactive and this might make sex dangerous. With the great majority of radiotherapy treatments this is not the case. The radiation does not stay in your body after your treatment session has ended. Where there is any radioactivity still in your body, as may be the case with some brachytherapy treatments, your doctors and therapists will always explain this to you and give you guidance.

One word of caution is that if you are a woman and you have had surgery or radiotherapy to your pelvis as part of your treatment before radiotherapy, then you should check how soon it will be safe for you to restart penetrative sex. Your specialist nurses will usually discuss this with you as part of their care during your treatment.

Although there is no medical reason why you should not continue your normal love life during your treatment, many people simply don't feel like it. This may be due to a number of things.

- *Tiredness*. Feeling tired and completely drained of energy is the most common of all the side effects of radiotherapy and most people just don't feel like having sex when they feel worn out.
- *Other side effects*. The radiotherapy may cause other side effects that are upsetting and just make you feel miserable. No one is likely to enjoy sex if they are feeling nauseated.
- *Anxiety*. Being worried about your cancer and its treatment is very understandable, and if you are feeling anxious then you are likely to be less keen on sex.
- *Depression*. Sometimes natural anxiety tips over into clinical depression, generally feeling low and lacking interest in things, including love-making.
- *The effects of the cancer*. If your cancer is still present then the illness itself may be making you feel unwell and switching off your interest.

Any or all of these things may affect your feelings about sex while you are having radiotherapy, and for some time afterwards.

The first, and most important, step in handling this change in your feelings is talking. And the most important person to talk to is your partner. Many people find that talking about sex, and in particular their own needs and emotions, is not easy. But letting your partner know what you are experiencing is essential, so that the two of you can reach a shared understanding of the way you are feeling. Talking may be hard, but it is far better than hiding your worries and concerns, or trying to pretend that things are normal when they are not.

Usually partners will be understanding, supportive and sympathetic. So that once you break the ice of bringing up the subject of sex, finding ways forward together to adapt to your altered desires and emotions should become easier, and you will at least have created a starting point from where you can work together to sort out any problems that your change in sexuality is causing in your relationship.

However, for some couples communication is more difficult, and even just starting to talk together about anything as sensitive as sex may be hard. If this is the case, then counselling may be a help. A trained counsellor might well be able to overcome the reservations, inhibitions or anxieties that are holding back an open discussion of the subject, and not only help sort out what the problems are, but pave the way to finding solutions to them. Quite a few hospitals have counsellors available for their cancer patients, and there are also sources of help outside the NHS.

Once this background awareness of the situation has been established, you can go on to look at ways of coping with it. The most likely difficulty is a mismatch in desire, with the person who is having treatment feeling less sexy, while their partner's libido remains much the same. This is very natural for both parties and neither of you should be guilty about the way you are feeling. Once again, talking helps to reach an understanding that your physical desires are different, and that that difference is entirely reasonable. From that basis of acceptance of difference, you can begin to sort out how to handle the situation. The solutions will be different for different people. They might include an agreed abstinence, a period of celibacy till you both feel the time is right, or you might adjust your relationship to one of hugs, caresses and cuddles, showing your love physically without actual sex; or you might change your approach to sex, with a greater emphasis on things like touching, stroking and masturbation, rather than penetrative sex, or changes in position that make actual intercourse more relaxed and less tiring.

These adjustments can only be made by the two of you, and can only be achieved by talking and understanding. There are no rights and wrongs, no set rules, for how the sexual dynamics of a couple should change at these times, so finding out what works for you is the right answer rather than thinking there is some magic formula that you ought to try and follow.

Another physical factor that may influence your sex life is a change in your physical appearance or body image. This is most likely to be due to treatment you have had before radiotherapy, such as an operation like a mastectomy, where a breast has been removed, or bowel surgery that has left you with a colostomy. Once again, changes in body image affect everyone differently. Some people take them in their stride and feel that a change in their physical appearance has little or nothing to do with the real 'them' and makes little or no difference to the person they are, whereas, at the other extreme, some people feel completely devastated by the change. Similarly, the effect on partners can be very variable, with some feeling that a mere physical change has not altered the person they know and love, while others find the altered appearance more unsettling. Talking is the key to adjusting to this situation. The likelihood is that if you are worried, your partner will be able to offer you reassurance that 'you' are still the person they love and care for and that any change in your appearance makes no difference to those feelings.

In terms of physical intimacy, you or your partner might at first find that change off-putting. The probability is that, after talking about it, that feeling would lessen or disappear. But if it remains a tension, then it might be possible to get round it by adjusting the technique of your love-making so that you could hide the change, covering the area, or keeping certain bits of clothing on during intercourse. Sometimes these new ways of love-making actually lead not only to a renewal of desire, but an increase in enjoyment with the novelty of the new approaches to sex.

This section has tended to look at the problem relating to sexuality during and after radiotherapy. But although there will always be times when sex does not appeal, many people find that they can continue not only to have sex during the time of their treatment, but to carry on enjoying it. And if you feel like it, then there is no reason at all why you should not go ahead and have some fun!

Friends and neighbours

Having cancer, and having radiotherapy, can sometimes alter day-to-day relationships with friends and neighbours. On occasions, the changes can be for the better, sometimes for the worse. If there is a problem, then it usually comes down to communication, with either them not understanding your feelings or you not under-standing theirs.

Everyone handles their cancer and its treatment differently. You may feel most comfortable by trying to keep things as much to yourself as possible, not sharing your thoughts and feelings with other people, carrying on as near normal as possible. If this is a positive way forward for you, if it helps you feel empowered and in control of your situation, and makes you feel stronger, then that is fine. But if you are simply trying to put a brave face on things because you don't want to burden other people, feeling that if you do so you will be letting yourself down or giving in, then think again because so often sharing your worries and talking things through can be very helpful and supportive. Bringing anxieties and stresses into the open can make them seem far less troubling than bottling them up.

Similarly, friends and neighbours may feel uncertain about how to handle your situation. Should they rush in with offers of help? Should they ask you about how you are getting on, or should they avoid the subject and pretend nothing is happening? They may worry that visiting you will make you tired or expose you to the risk of minor infections. They may even worry that they could 'catch' cancer from you (which, of course, can never happen).

There are many ways of coping and it is down to you how you decide to handle this situation. If you want to try and carry on as normally as possible, and feel you cope best in that way, then let people know. Equally, if you are happy to talk about what is happening to you, and if sharing some or all of what you are going through makes life easier, then again let those around you know that you would welcome their questions and concerns. Or you may just want the practical support they can give: help with the shopping, lifts to and from the hospital, looking after the children once in a while, without the emotional involvement of talking about your thoughts and feelings. But however you want to deal with things, it will make life easier for them – and, more importantly, for you – if you let them know.

Telling them might be something you find quite straightforward, or you might feel it is difficult and that it is just one more burden to deal with. If this is the case, then getting your partner, or someone close to you in the family, to have a word with friends and neighbours for you could solve the problem.

Useful addresses

There are many organizations that offer help and advice to people with cancer, and a lot of these cover just one particular type of cancer. The short list that follows gives details of the main providers of general information; and they all give details of, and have links to, many other sources of help that you may find useful.

These organizations will also give you more ideas for further reading – many of them have lists of books, booklets and other reading material, that are updated on a regular basis.

Cancerbackup
3 Bath Place
Rivington Street
London EC2A 3JR
Freephone Helpline: 0808 800 1234
Website: www.cancerbackup.org.uk

Cancerbackup is a comprehensive information service for patients. It offers a telephone helpline to specially trained cancer nurses, who can give advice on all aspects of cancer and the relevant treatment needed. Cancerbackup also produces nearly 70 booklets, and more than 200 factsheets, again covering all aspects of cancer. There are also more than 1200 questions and answers about cancer on its website (the website also has the texts of all the booklets and factsheets, and links to many other useful organizations).

Cancer Research UK
PO Box 123
Lincoln's Inn Fields
London WC2A 3PX
Tel.: 020 7121 6699
Website: www.cancerresearchuk.org

As well as funding research on cancer, this organization has a website (<www.cancerhelp.org.uk>) that gives information about all the different types of cancer and their treatment, as well as a comprehensive list of clinical trials currently in progress.

DIPEx (Database of Individual Patient Experiences)
Website: www.dipex.org

This website covers a number of different illnesses, but has an extensive section on cancer. This not only gives some background information on various types of cancer, but has lots of stories from people who have had cancer and gone through chemotherapy.

Macmillan Cancer Support
89 Albert Embankment
London SE1 7UQ
Tel.: 0808 808 2020
Website: www.macmillan.org.uk

In addition to funding cancer nursing services, this organization provides a number of publications on cancer, including a useful booklet on benefits and financial help for cancer patients (all listed on their website). The website also has useful information on various aspects of cancer, and includes a directory of local cancer support groups, and patients' stories about cancer.

The Royal College of Radiologists
Website: www.rcr.ac.uk

The College website has a virtual guide to a radiotherapy department. Click on 'virtual hospital' and then click on 'oncology' to find the guide.

Index